Using and
Understanding
Medical Statistics

David E. Matthews
Vernon T. Farewell

Using and Understanding Medical Statistics

2nd, revised edition

28 figures and 82 tables, 1988

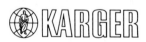

Basel · München · Paris · London · NewYork · NewDelhi · Singapore · Tokyo · Sydney

David Edward Matthews

BA, MA (Western Ontario), PhD (London);
Associate Professor, Department of Statistics and Actuarial Science,
University of Waterloo, Waterloo, Ontario, Canada

Vernon T. Farewell

B. Math, M. Math (Waterloo), PhD (London);
Professor, Departments of Statistics and Actuarial Science and Health Studies,
University of Waterloo, Waterloo, Ontario, Canada

© Copyright 1988 by S. Karger AG, P.O. Box, CH–4009 Basel (Switzerland)
Printed in Switzerland by Thür AG Offsetdruck, Pratteln
ISBN 3–8055–4719–6

To Nancy and Jane

Contents

Contents

Preface to the First Edition

The origins of this book can be traced to a short course which was offered in the autumn of 1980 to medical researchers at the Fred Hutchinson Cancer Research Center. The syllabus for that course was drawn up to meet the specific needs of those researchers. After re-examining the material we had presented, we felt that the content of the course and the approach we had adopted were different from their counterparts in familiar introductory books on statistics, even those which were written specifically for medical researchers. Unsolicited comments from course participants encouraged us to develop and expand our approach instead of filing the assorted tables and handouts. And so, through additions, deletions and numerous revisions, the final product haltingly took shape and assumed its present form.

Our aim now, as in 1980, is quite simple: to describe the statistical methodology which frequently is found in published medical research, particularly those papers concerned with chronic diseases. This presentation introduces, in some detail, fundamental statistical notions which are common to nearly every method of analyzing data – for example, significance tests. From these foundations we direct our attention to more advanced methods of analysis. In order to avoid excessive complexity in the initial chapters, we rely on the promise of bigger and better things to come to motivate the selected topics we choose to discuss. Nonetheless, there is sufficient introductory detail that we feel obliged to ask our readers to exercise more patience and endurance than most introductions to medical statistics require. We are convinced that solid beginnings are essential to any *useful* discussion of the important, more advanced methodology which frequently is used in modern medical research.

We have written for the motivated reader who is willing to invest a little time and effort in understanding statistical methods. On the other hand, our constant goal has been to write a book which could be read fairly easily in installments. We hope that most chapters represent a single evening's reading. Although one might decide to devote a little more time to some of the details, it should then be possible to tackle the next chapter. We shall be pleased if we have succeeded in achieving this goal; however, we do not wish to be regarded as competing with alternative evening reading which may be more interesting or exciting!

Except, perhaps, for an over-emphasis on chronic diseases, we believe that a medical student who understands the contents of this book will be well-informed regarding medical statistics. Whether medical students, who often regard statistics as an unnecessary evil, should and can be adequately motivated to master this material is an open question. We have not attempted to provide this motivation ourselves. In our view, the most persuasive arguments on behalf of the subject will always be those advanced by medical researchers who have themselves established a use for statistical analysis which does not depend on the editorial policy of medical journals.

The final preparation of this manuscript took place while one of us (V.F.) was visiting the Department of Biomathematics at the University of Oxford, and the other (D.M.) was visiting the Department of Medical Statistics and Epidemiology at the London School of Hygiene and Tropical Medicine. We want to thank Professors *Peter Armitage* and *Michael Healy* for making these visits possible. We are also greatly indebted to Mrs. *Joy Hoggarth* at the Fred Hutchinson Cancer Research Center for her superb preparation of the manuscript. She was greatly handicapped by being more than 5,000 miles from the authors.

An early version of this book was read by Dr. *G.J. D'Angio* of the Children's Hospital of Philadelphia; his helpful comments and criticisms had a significant influence on the final manuscript. We thank him for this and, in general, for his unwavering support of statistics in medical research. It is our hope that this book will help other investigators to develop a similar appreciation for the value of medical statistics.

D.E. Matthews
V.T. Farewell

Preface to the Second Edition

Slightly less than four years have elapsed since the preface to the first edition was written. In the meantime, we have been surprised, and pleased, by the response to the first edition. The letters and comments which we have received from readers and reviewers on several continents have brought us much satisfaction. Suggestions and criticisms have helped us to understand specific topics where the first edition failed to meet the goals which we had established. Despite our best intentions, there were inevitable errors in the first edition which we were anxious to correct. Consequently, when the publisher inquired about the possibility of a revised edition, we realized that it would be an opportunity to rectify both kinds of flaws simultaneously.

How do the two editions differ? Apart from minor corrections to Table 3.4 and the elimination of errors which appear to be randomly distributed through the chapters, the principal differences may be found in the second half of the book. The example in chapter 10 has been changed to one which we believe suits better the purpose we intend to achieve. Sections have been added to chapters 11, 12 and 14 which treat topics that were previously omitted. In some ways, these additions reflect the changing face of medical statistics, and the clinical investigations in which statistical methods play an important role. However, the major difference between the editions is the addition of chapter 16, which concerns epidemiological studies. The topics treated in the final chapter illustrate just how much the use of sophisticated statistical analysis has permeated the recent practice of epidemiology. At the same time, this new chapter knits together the fabric of the book, drawing on methods which we have introduced in previous chapters to analyze data from various epidemiological studies. In that respect, chapter 16 does what no chapter in the first edition was able to do. We hope its inclusion in the second edition will help all readers, even those whose main interest is not directed towards epidemiology, to integrate their understanding and extend their appreciation for the use of statistical methods in medical research.

We are grateful to Ms *Lynda Clarke* in the Department of Statistics and Actuarial Science at the University of Waterloo. Her skill and cheerful co-operation made light work of all our changes in the process of preparing the revised manuscript.

D.E. Matthews
V.T. Farewell

1 Basic Concepts

1.1. Introduction

A brief glance through almost any recently published medical journal will show that statistical methods are playing an increasingly visible role in modern medical research. At the very least, most research papers quote (at least) one 'p-value' to underscore the 'significance' of the results which the authors wish to communicate. At the same time, a growing number of papers are now presenting the results of relatively sophisticated, 'multi-factor' statistical analyses of complex sets of medical data. This proliferation in the use of statistical methods has also been paralleled by the increased involvement of professionally trained statisticians in medical research as consultants to and collaborators with the medical researchers themselves.

The primary purpose of this book is to provide medical researchers with sufficient understanding to enable them to read, intelligently, statistical methods and discussion appearing in medical journals. At the same time, we have tried to provide the means for researchers to undertake the simpler analyses on their own, if this is their wish. And by presenting statistics from this perspective, we hope to extend and improve the common base of understanding which is necessary whenever medical researchers and statisticians interact.

It seems obvious to us that statisticians involved in medical research need to have some understanding of the related medical knowledge. We also believe that in order to benefit from statistical advice, medical researchers require some understanding of the subject of statistics. This first chapter provides a brief introduction to some of the terms and symbols which recur throughout the book. It also establishes what statisticians talk about (random variables, probability distributions) and how they talk about these concepts (standard notation). We are very aware that this material is difficult to motivate; it seems so distant from the core and purpose of medical statistics. Nevertheless, 'these dry bones' provide a skeleton which allows the rest of the book to be more precise about statistics and medical research than would otherwise be possible. Therefore, we urge the reader to forbear with these beginnings, and read beyond the end of chapter 1 to see whether we do not put flesh onto these dry bones.

1.2. Random Variables, Probability Distributions and Some Standard Notation

Most statistical work is based on the concept of a random variable. This is a quantity which, theoretically, may assume a wide variety of actual values, although in any particular instance we only observe a single value. Measurements are common examples of random variables; take the weight of a patient, for example. The actual weight of a particular patient is naturally subject to a degree of variability due to the physical constraints of the measuring scale, and repeated measurements of the patient's weight would almost certainly result in similar, but not identical, measurements. Thus, a statistician might refer to the random variable representing the weight of the patient. Another example of a random variable might be the systolic blood pressure reading; for a single individual, this measurement can be quite variable.

To represent a particular random variable, statisticians generally use an upper case Roman letter, say X or Y. The particular value which this random variable represents in a specific case is often denoted by the corresponding lower case Roman letter, say x or y. The probability distribution (usually shortened to the distribution) of any random variable can be thought of as a specification of all possible numerical values of the random variable, together with an indication of the frequency with which each numerical value occurs in the population of interest.

It is common statistical shorthand to use subscripted letters – x_1, x_2, ..., x_n, for example – to specify a set of observed values of the random variable X. The corresponding notation for the set of random variables is X_i, i = 1, 2, ..., n, where X_i indicates that the random variable of interest is labelled X and the symbols i = 1, 2, ..., n specify the possible values of the subscripts on X. Similarly, using n as the final subscript in the set simply indicates that the size of the set may vary from one instance to another, but in each particular instance it will be a fixed number.

Subscripted letters constitute extremely useful notation for the statistician, who must specify precise formulae which will subsequently be applied in particular situations which vary enormously. At this point it is also convenient to introduce the use of Σ, the upper case Greek letter sigma. In mathematics, Σ represents summation. To specify the sum $X_1 + X_2 + X_3$ we would simply write $\sum_{i=1}^{3} X_i$. This expression specifies that the subscript i should take the values 1, 2 and 3 in turn, and we should sum the resulting variables. For a fixed but unspecified number of variables, say n, the sum $X_1 + X_2 + ... + X_n$ would be represented by $\sum_{i=1}^{n} X_i$.

A set of values $x_1, x_2, ..., x_n$ is called a sample from the population of all possible occurrences of X. In general, statistical procedures which use such a sample assume that it is a random sample from the population. The random sample assumption is imposed to ensure that the characteristics of the sample reflect those of the entire population, of which the sample is often only a small part.

There are two types of random variables. If we ignore certain technicalities, a discrete random variable is commonly defined as one for which we can write down all its possible values and their corresponding frequencies of occurrence. In contrast, continuous random variables are measured on an interval scale, and the variable can assume any value on the scale. Of course, the instruments which we use to measure experimental quantities (e.g., blood pressure, acid concentration, weight, height, etc.) have a finite resolution, but it is convenient to suppose, in such situations, that this limitation does not prevent us from observing any plausible measurement. Furthermore, the notation which statisticians have adopted to represent all possible values belonging to a given interval is to enclose the endpoints of the interval in parentheses. Thus, (a, b) specifies the set of all possible values between a and b, and the symbolic statement '$a < X < b$' means that the random variable X takes a value in the interval specified by (a, b).

The probability distribution of a random variable is often illustrated by means of a histogram or bar graph. This is a picture which indicates how frequently each value of the random variable occurs, either in a sample or in the corresponding population. If the random variable is discrete, the picture is generally a simple one to draw and to understand. Figure 1.1a shows a histogram for the random variable, S, which represents the sum of the showing faces of two fair dice. Notice that there are exactly 11 possible values for S. In contrast to this situation, the histogram for a continuous random variable, say systolic blood pressure, X, is somewhat more difficult to draw and to understand. One such histogram is presented in Figure 1.1b. Since the picture is intended to show both the possible values of X and also the frequency with which they arise, each rectangular block in the graph has an area equal to the proportion of the sample represented by all outcomes belonging to the interval on the base of the block. This has the effect of equating frequency, or probability of occurrence, with area and is known as the 'area = probability' equation for continuous random variables.

To a statistician, histograms are simply an approximate picture of the mathematical way of describing the distribution of a continuous random variable. A more accurate representation of the distribution is obtained by using the equation of a curve which can best be thought of as a 'smooth histogram'; such a curve is called a probability density function. A more convenient term, and one which we intend to use, is probability curve.

Figure 1.2a shows the probability curve, or smooth histogram, for the continuous random variable, X, which we used above to represent systolic blood pressure. This curve is, in fact, the probability curve which has the characteristic shape and equation known as a 'normal distribution'. Random variables which have a normal distribution will recur in subsequent chapters, and we intend to explain their properties and uses in more detail at that time. For the present, however, we want to concentrate on the concept of the area = probability equation. Figure 1.2b shows two shaded areas. One is the area below the curve and above the interval (110, 130). Recall that the symbol (110, 130) represents all blood pressure measurements between 110 and 130. Because of the area = probability equation for the continuous random variable X, the shaded area above (110, 130) corresponds, pictorially, to the probability that systolic blood pressure in the population is between 110 and 130. This area can be calculated mathematically, and in this particular example the value is 0.323. To represent this calculation in a symbolic statement we would write $\Pr(110 < X < 130) = 0.323$; the equation states that the probability that X, a systolic blood pressure measurement in the population, is between 110 and 130 is equal to 0.323.

The second shaded area in Figure 1.2b is the area below the probability curve corresponding to values of X in the interval (165, ∞), i.e., the probability that a systolic blood pressure measurement in the population exceeds 165. By means of certain calculations we can determine that, for this specific example, the probability that systolic blood pressure exceeds 165 is 0.023; the concise mathematical description of this calculation is simply $\Pr(X > 165) = 0.023$.

Although the probability curve makes it easy to picture the equality of area and probability, it is of little direct use for actually calculating probabilities since areas cannot be read directly from a picture or sketch. Instead, we need a related function called the cumulative probability curve. Figure 1.3 presents the cumulative probability curve for the normal distribution shown

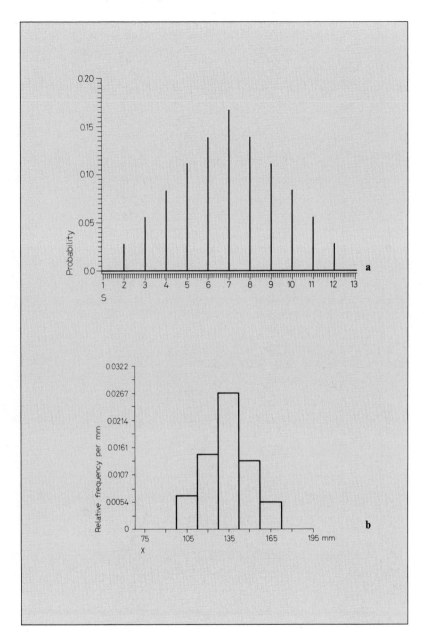

Fig. 1.1. Histograms of random variables. **a** The discrete random variable, S, representing the sum of the showing faces for two fair dice. **b** Fifty observations on the continuous random variable, X, representing systolic blood pressure.

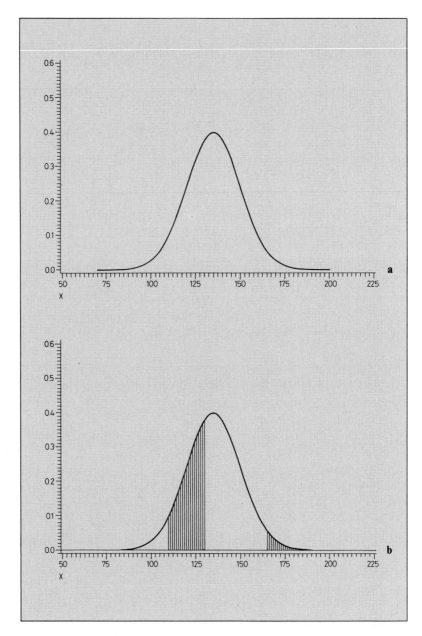

Fig. 1.2. A probability curve for the continuous random variable, X, representing systolic blood pressure. **a** As a smooth histogram. **b** With shaded areas corresponding to Pr(110 < X < 130) and Pr(X > 165).

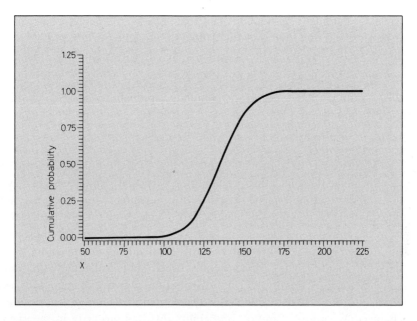

Fig. 1.3. The cumulative probability curve for the random variable, X, representing systolic blood pressure.

in Figure 1.2a. The horizontal axis represents the possible values of the random variable X; the vertical axis is a probability scale with values ranging from zero to one. The cumulative probability curve specifies, for each value a, say, on the horizontal axis, the probability that the random variable X takes a value which is at most a, i.e., $Pr(X \leq a)$. This probability is precisely the area below the probability curve corresponding to values of X in the interval $(-\infty, a)$. In particular, if $a = \infty$, i.e., $Pr(-\infty < X < \infty)$, the value of the cumulative probability curve is one, indicating that X is certain to assume a value in the interval $(-\infty, \infty)$. In fact, this result is a necessary property of all cumulative probability curves, and is equivalent to the statement that the area under any probability curve is always equal to one.

Clearly, a cumulative probability curve is more useful than the corresponding probability curve for actually calculating probabilities. For example, since the area under the probability curve always equals one, it follows that

$$Pr(X > a) = 1 - Pr(X \leq a).$$

Thus, the cumulative probability curve can be used to calculate the probability corresponding to the interval (a, ∞). And for the interval (a, b), where a and b are two specific values, it is fairly easy to show that

$$\Pr(a < X < b) = \Pr(X < b) - \Pr(X \leqslant a);$$

this is simply a difference of the cumulative probability curve evaluated at the two points a and b.

Comment:

Most readers have probably noticed that §1.2 did not contain any specific formulae for calculating probabilities, particularly in the case of continuous random variables. The reason for this is simple. More frequently than not, the calculations are sufficiently formidable, numerically, that statisticians have prepared standardized tables to make the evaluation of probabilities relatively simple. These tables, which often are tabulations of the cumulative probability curve, are generally called statistical tables; the values which we quoted for the normal distribution shown in Figure 1.2b were obtained from a statistical table for the normal distribution. In subsequent chapters, as various common probability distributions arise in the exposition, we will discuss how to use the relevant statistical table.

1.3. Characteristics of a Distribution: Mean, Median and Variance

If we wish to be absolutely precise about the distribution of a certain random variable, say X, then we must specify the equation of the probability curve if it is a continuous random variable, or the values of X and the probability with which they occur if X is a discrete random variable. However, if we only wish to indicate something about the distribution of X in general terms, it often suffices to specify the location and spread of the distribution of X. In common, everyday terms this is equivalent to the two usual answers to the question 'Where is X's office?'. If you wish to be precise you would answer 'X's office is Room 703 at 1024 Columbia Street, in the Cabrini Tower'. On the other hand, if you were only planning to offer a general answer to the question you would reply 'X's office is on Capitol Hill'.

1.3.1. Location

A measure of location for the distribution of a random variable, X, should tell us the value which is roughly central, in some sense, to the range of values where X is regularly observed to occur. The most common measure

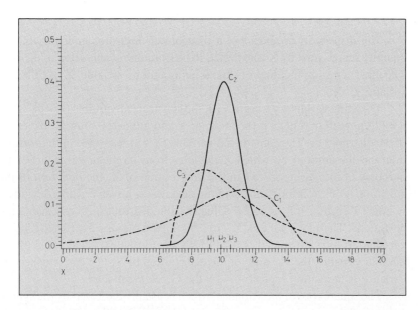

Fig. 1.4. Three probability curves, C_1, C_2 and C_3, having the same median (10) but different means μ_1, μ_2 and μ_3, respectively.

of location used by statisticians is the mean or expected value of X; this is denoted by the symbol E(X). If we think, for a moment, of a probability associated with the distribution of X as mass, then the mean value, E(X), is located at the center of mass. The Greek letter μ is often used to represent E(X).

A second measure of location is the median value of X. Most readers will recognize the median as the measure of location which is commonly used in the medical literature. The median of X is that particular value which equally divides the probability in the distribution of X, i.e., with probability ½ an observed value of X will exceed the median and with probability ½ an observed value will not exceed the median.

In general, the median of X and the mean, E(X), are different because the median is less influenced by extreme values of X which might occur than is E(X). However, if the distribution of X below the median is a mirror image of the upper half of the distribution, then the distribution is said to be symmetric and the median and mean will coincide. To illustrate some of the differences between the mean and the median, Figure 1.4 shows three probability curves which have the same median but different means.

1.3.2. Spread

The dispersion or spread of a distribution indicates how variable the quantity represented by X is expected to be from one observation to the next. The most common measure of spread for a random variable, X, is called the variance of X.

To define variance we begin with the constructed variable $(X - \mu)$, where $\mu = E(X)$; recall that $E(X)$ is the mean of X and indicates, roughly, the center of the distribution. The constructed variable $(X - \mu)$ measures both the direction and the amount by which X deviates from its mean value μ. For the purposes of measuring spread in the distribution of X, the direction of this deviation is of less importance than the magnitude; however, large deviations in either direction influence the spread of the distribution more than small deviations. Therefore, we use $(X - \mu)^2$, the square of our constructed random variable, to indicate spread and call $E\{(X - \mu)^2\}$, the expected value of this random variable, the variance of the distribution of X. For convenience, the variance is frequently represented by the Greek symbol σ^2.

The square root of the variance, which is usually indicated by the symbol σ, is called the standard error or standard deviation of the distribution of X. By specifying the mean, μ, and standard error, σ, for the distribution of X, we are providing an approximate or general description of the entire distribution. But to evaluate probabilities for a distribution, or to perform other calculations, we need more specific information than just the mean and standard error. For accurate calculations we also require the equation of the cumulative probability curve or suitable tables. However, these are details which we intend to discuss in later chapters.

Too often the beginnings of any subject will kill the enthusiasm of the most eager reader. However, now that the groundwork has been done, we can proceed to discuss some of the basic procedures which statisticians have developed. The first of these which we will consider, and therefore the subject of chapter 2, is called a test of significance.

2 Tests of Significance

2.1. Introduction

Among the statistical methods employed in medical research, tests of significance enjoy a pre-eminent position. Whether this importance is justified could be, and sometimes is, a matter for heated debate. In this chapter, however, it is our intention to identify the features which are common to all tests of significance in order that particular tests which we will consider in subsequent chapters may be readily understood.

A test of significance is a statistical procedure by which one determines the degree to which collected data are consistent with a specific hypothesis which is under investigation. There is a sense in which the process of arriving at a medical diagnosis may be compared to a test of significance. Consider the general practitioner treating a patient who has recently become ill. The patient's physical appearance and brief description of the symptoms prompts the physician to compile a list of perhaps three or four possible causes; each cause is a hypothesis of interest. Next, the physician uses knowledge and experience to examine the patient. The examination results in observed data concerning the patient's present condition. Finally, the physician evaluates the situation, determining the degree to which the observed data are consistent with each possible cause. The diagnosis identifies the single cause, or hypothesis, to which the weight of medical evidence points.

As we mentioned before, a significance test is quite similar to the diagnostic process described above. Of course, there are differences which are important. Nevertheless, the physician and the statistician are each interested in assessing the degree to which observed data are consistent with a specific hypothesis. In statistical parlance, the result of the evaluation process is called the significance level ('p-value') of the data with respect to the hypothesis. Of course, there are assumptions and calculations which are an implicit part of the evaluation process. In fact, there are six features which are common to all significance tests, and §2.3 is chiefly a discussion of these features. But first, we propose to consider a specific example, and to explain the assumptions and arguments which give rise to the significance level of a test and the resulting conclusion.

2.2. An Example

Thomas et al. [1983] discuss relapse patterns in irradiated Wilms' tumor patients. In particular, they describe a review of radiotherapy records which indicated that 23 out of 259 patients were judged to have been treated with a radiation field of inadequate size. An obvious hypothesis of interest is the suggestion that inadequate radiotherapy is associated with a higher risk of relapse in the operative site. Subsequent investigation of these 259 patients revealed that there were four relapses in the operative site, two of which occurred in the 23 patients who received inadequate radiotherapy. The data may be concisely presented in a summary table containing two rows and two columns (see Table 2.1); tables of this form are usually called 2×2 contingency tables.

A major purpose of this study of 259 patients was to determine whether inadequate radiotherapy is associated with a higher risk of relapse in the operative site. If we examine the data, we see that the relapse rate among patients whose field size was adequate was 2/236 (0.9%), whereas the corresponding figure for patients who received inadequate radiotherapy was 2/23 (8.7%). If *Thomas* et al. were only interested in the hypothesis concerning relapse in the operative site for the 259 patients studied, then the data indicate that inadequate field size is associated with an elevated relapse rate in those 23 patients. However, this is not the question which the researchers want to answer. They are interested in the population of patients who are treated for Wilms' tumor. The 259 patients in the study constitute a sample from that population. On the basis of the data collected from the sample, *Thomas* et al. wish to infer whether the relapse rate in the operative site is higher for all patients in the population who receive inadequate radiotherapy.

In order to arrive at any conclusions regarding the hypothesis of an elevated risk of relapse based on the sample data, we must assume that the sample is truly representative of the population in all pertinent respects. However, even if we assume that this is true, how should the results of the study be interpreted? Should we conclude that the sample relapse rates (0.009 and 0.087) are the same as the population relapse rates, and therefore inadequate field size is associated with a ten-fold increase in the risk of relapse? Surely not! After all, the sample size is fixed at 259 patients, 23 of whom received inadequate radiotherapy, and only four relapses in the operative site were observed. If we adjust the numbers in the four cells of the 2×2 table, always taking care to maintain the same row and column totals, then we see

Table 2.1. A 2×2 contingency table summarizing the data described in *Thomas* et al. [1983]

	Field size too small	Field size adequate	Total
Operative site relapse	2	2	4
No operative site relapse	21	234	255
Total	23	236	259

that only five different 2×2 tables could possibly be observed in a study of 259 patients with these relapse and treatment totals. These five tables (labelled 0 through 4 for convenience) are displayed in Figure 2.1; notice that the label for each 2×2 table corresponds to the number in the upper left-hand corner. The sample relapse rates for each of these tables are indicated in Table 2.2.

Table 2.2 illustrates the folly of assuming that sample relapse rates are the same as population relapse rates. Quite obviously, the fixed study totals (259 patients, 4 relapses and 23 patients receiving inadequate radiotherapy) severely restrict the set of possible sample relapse rates that may be observed to exactly five pairs of values.

This problem with sample relapse rates suggests that perhaps we should redirect our attention from the sample to the population. Clearly, there is a population relapse rate, r_1 say, for patients who received adequate radiotherapy, and there is a second relapse rate, r_2 say, for patients whose radiotherapy was inadequate. The hypothesis which *Thomas* et al. wish to investigate is whether or not these relapse rates are the same, i.e., whether $r_1 = r_2$ or $r_1 \neq r_2$. If r_1 and r_2 are identical, or very similar, then we might expect this similarity to be reflected in the observed data, to the extent that the sample size, number of relapses and treatment totals permit. On the other hand, if r_1 and r_2 are quite different, then we would expect the data to reflect this difference, again, as the numbers permit.

If we suppose that r_1 and r_2 are the same, then a natural estimate of the common relapse rate $r = r_1 = r_2$, say, is $4/259 = 0.015$, the overall relapse rate in the sample. Of course, r is unlikely to be exactly 0.015; nevertheless, if our sample is representative of the population, r should be fairly close to the observed relapse rate. And if 0.015 is close to r, the relapse rate in the population of Wilms' tumor patients, then among the 23 who received inadequate radiotherapy we would expect to observe approximately $23 \times 0.015 = $

Table 0

	Field size too small	Field size adequate	Total
Operative site relapse	0	4	4
No operative site relapse	23	232	255
Total	23	236	259

Table 1

1	3	4
22	233	255
23	236	259

Table 2

2	2	4
21	234	255
23	236	259

Table 3

3	1	4
20	235	255
23	236	259

Table 4

4	0	4
19	236	255
23	236	259

Fig. 2.1. The five possible 2×2 tables with fixed marginal totals 4, 255, 23 and 236.

0.355 relapses in the operative site. From this perspective we realize that there is an obvious ranking for Tables 0 through 4, based on the observed number of relapses among the 23 patients who received inadequate radiotherapy. If the population relapse rates are the same, i.e., $r_1 = r_2$, then Table 0 is most consistent with that situation, Table 1 is less consistent than Table 0 and so on; Table 4 is clearly the least consistent of all five possible sample outcomes. To express this idea in a somewhat different way, we might say that, if $r_1 = r_2$, then we would be most inclined to expect Table 0 to result from the review of patient records, and least inclined to expect Table 4.

Once we have realized this fact, we have begun to develop an objective method of evaluating the degree of consistency between the data and the hypothesis of interest. Nevertheless, we still have a considerable distance to cover. For example, it should be clear that because the study patients are a

Table 2.2. Sample relapse rates in Tables 0 through 4

	Table #				
	0	1	2	3	4
Field size too small	0.0	0.044	0.087	0.130	0.174
Field size adequate	0.017	0.013	0.009	0.004	0.0

Table 2.3. The probability of observing each of Tables 0 through 4 if $r_1 = r_2$

	Table #					Total
	0	1	2	3	4	
Probability	0.6875	0.2715	0.0386	0.0023	0.0001	1.0000

sample from the population, and because sampling necessarily involves uncertainty, we cannot state conclusively that, if $r_1 = r_2$, the study records would not yield Table 4. Quite obviously, what we need now is an objective measure of how likely, or unlikely, each of Tables 0 through 4 would be if the relapse rates r_1 and r_2 are the same. And this is precisely what probability calculations can provide. If we assume, a priori, that $r_1 = r_2$, then it is fairly simple for a statistician to calculate the probability that in a sample of 259 patients, 23 of whom received inadequate radiotherapy and 4 of whom relapsed at the operative site, exactly 0 (or 1, 2, 3 or 4) patients who relapsed also received inadequate radiotherapy. Rather than labor over the details of these calculations, we have listed the probabilities in Table 2.3 and will defer the details to chapter 3.

The entries in Table 2.3 indicate that, if the population relapse rates for both groups of Wilms' tumor patients are the same, then samples of size 259 having the same relapse and treatment totals (4 and 23, respectively) are most likely to yield Table 0 and least likely to result in Table 4. However, each of the five tables might possibly occur in a particular sampling situation. Notice, also, that Table 2 (which was reported by *Thomas* et al.) is a relatively unlikely outcome if the equal relapse rates assumption is correct. If we consider all tables which are no more consistent with the hypothesis $r_1 = r_2$

Table 2.4. The two possible explanations for the observed result in the study of *Thomas* et al. [1983]

	Explanation 1	Explanation 2
Hypothesis	The relapse rates r_1, r_2 are the same (i.e., $r_1 = r_2$)	The relapse rates r_1, r_2 are different (i.e., $r_1 \neq r_2$)
Observed result	The observed difference in the sample relapse rates is due to sampling uncertainty (chance)	The observed difference in the sample relapse rates reflects the true difference between r_1 and r_2 in the population

than Table 2, i.e., Tables 2, 3 and 4, then by adding the corresponding probabilities we determine that data which are no more consistent with the hypothesis $r_1 = r_2$ than those which were observed (i.e., Tables 2, 3 and 4) could be expected to occur in approximately four studies out of every hundred having the same sample size (259), relapse and treatment totals (4, 23, respectively). It is this value, 0.041, the sum of the probabilities for Tables 2, 3 and 4, that statisticians call the significance level (p-value) of a test of the hypothesis $r_1 = r_2$.

At this point in the argument we pause to consider possible explanations for the observed result. Each explanation is based on a specific hypothesis about the population relapse rates. Clearly, to be satisfactory, an explanation should account for the significance level of the data. As Table 2.4 indicates, there are basically two explanations which account for the result observed in the sample of *Thomas* et al.

Clearly, we cannot determine which explanation, if either, is correct; this is beyond the realm of statistics. We cannot determine directly whether Explanation 1 is more likely since, if $r_1 \neq r_2$, we do not know how great is the actual difference in relapse rates. However, we do know that if Explanation 1 is correct, the significance level ($p = 0.04$) specifies how likely we would be to obtain a study sample which is no more consistent with the hypothesis of equal relapse rates than Table 2.

Which explanation is preferable, the first or the second? As a general rule in scientific research, the simplest description or model of a situation which is, at the same time, consistent with the available evidence is preferred. On this basis, Explanation 1 usually would be selected, a priori, because it does not involve a relapse rate which depends on the radiotherapy received. However, if we adopt Explanation 1, then we are also choosing to account for the observed difference in sample relapse rates on the basis of sampling uncertainty. We have calculated that such discrepancies would occur in at most four studies out of every hundred of a similar size. Statisticians normally suggest that when the significance level associated with the simpler explanation is very small, it is justifiable to conclude that the simpler explanation is not consistent with the evidence at hand; instead, the more complicated explanation should be adopted. Therefore, since the significance level of the data of *Thomas* et al. with respect to the hypothesis of equal relapse rates is relatively small (p = 0.04), we conclude from an analysis of the study records that the weight of evidence contradicts the hypothesis that $r_1 = r_2$, i.e., Explanation 2 is preferred.

2.3. Common Features of Significance Tests

The preceding example provides a valuable introduction to the general topic of significance tests. The purpose of a significance test is to determine the degree of consistency between a specific hypothesis, represented by H say, and a set of data. In most cases, H is a simple description of some aspect of a particular population and the collected data are obtained from a sample drawn from the population. While the sample is thought to be representative of the population, it is clear that a different sample would give rise to a different set of data. There are always two fairly obvious explanations for the observed results:

I   The hypothesis H is true and sampling uncertainty (chance) is the reason for the observed result.

II   The hypothesis H is false and the difference between the true situation and H is the reason for the observed result.

The objective measure which is used to evaluate the degree to which the data are consistent with the hypothesis H is a probability calculation of the sampling uncertainty referred to in Explanation I. If we assume H is true, we can calculate how likely, or unlikely, the outcome observed in the sample would be. If the outcome is likely (normally, this is thought to be the case when the significance level is at least 0.05, i.e., $p \geqslant 0.05$) then we have meager evidence, at best, for concluding that the data are inconsistent with H. However, if the outcome is unlikely when H is true (normally, this is thought to be the case when the significance level is less than 0.05, i.e., $p < 0.05$), then both I and II become plausible explanations. Provided the sampling procedure has been carefully designed to guard against gross defects, as the significance level (p-value) decreases we become less inclined to favor I, preferring II as the more plausible explanation for the apparent inconsistency between the data and the specific hypothesis H.

In summary, a significance test assumes that a specific hypothesis, H, about a population is true and compares the outcome observed in the sample with all other possible outcomes which sampling uncertainty might have generated. To carry out a test of significance, then, the following are necessary:

(1) A hypothesis about the population, usually referred to as H_0 (the null hypothesis). In the example discussed in §2.2, H_0 was the assumption that the population relapse rates, r_1 and r_2, were equal.

(2) Data from the population. These are obtained from a random sample and are usually summarized in the form of the observed value of a suitable test statistic. In the sample obtained by *Thomas* et al. [1983] the test statistic was the number of patients who had received inadequate radiotherapy and who had subsequently relapsed in the operative site; its value in the sample was 2.

(3) A set of comparable events of which the outcome observed in the sample is only one possibility. In the example of §2.2, the five possible 2×2 tables displayed in Figure 2.1 constitute the set of comparable events.

(4) The probability distribution of the test statistic (see 2), based on the assumptions that the null hypothesis, H_0, is true and the sampling uncertainty is random. For the example we discussed in §2.2, this probability distribution is displayed in Table 2.3.

(5) A ranking of all possible outcomes in the set of comparable events (see 3) according to their consistency with the null hypothesis H_0. In the example from *Thomas* et al. we ranked Tables 0 through 4 as follows:

	Most consistent with H_0			Least consistent with H_0
Table # 0	1	2	3	4

This ranking was based on the probability distribution displayed in Table 2.3.

(6) A calculation of the probability that sampling uncertainty (chance) would produce an outcome no more consistent with the null hypothesis, H_0, than the outcome which actually was observed (see 2). This probability is

called the significance level of the data with respect to H_0. In the example of §2.2, the significance level of the data with respect to the hypothesis of equal relapse rates was 0.041, the probability of obtaining Tables 2, 3 or 4.

Many tests of significance for standard situations have been devised by statisticians, and the items outlined in (1)–(6) above have been specified. Often, all that a researcher must do in a particular circumstance is to select an appropriate test, evaluate the prescribed test statistic using the collected data, calculate the significance level (p-value) of the data with respect to the null hypothesis, H_0, and draw an appropriate conclusion.

In succeeding chapters, we will describe particular tests of significance which are basic to medical statistics. In general, these chapters adopt a more relaxed presentation of specific significance tests than we have undertaken in this chapter. The particular test which we discussed in §2.2 is known as Fisher's test for 2×2 contingency tables. This test is sufficiently useful to justify a presentation in more general terms. In addition, since the specific details of the example in §2.2 are now familiar ground, a discussion of Fisher's test should ease the transition of any hesitant reader onto the new aspects of well-known territory which we shall introduce in chapter 3.

3 Fisher's Test for 2 × 2 Contingency Tables

3.1. Introduction

A surprising amount of the data gathered in medical research is binary in nature, that is, it belongs to one of only two possible outcomes. For example, patients treated for Wilms' tumor either relapse in the operative site or they do not. For this reason, the methods which statisticians have devised for analyzing binary data frequently find a natural application in medical research. Data which are binary usually can be summarized conveniently in a 2 × 2 contingency table such as the one discussed in §2.2. In these situations, it is natural to ask whether the two binary classification schemes, represented by the rows and columns of the 2 × 2 table, are associated in the population. If we assume that no such association exists, then Fisher's test determines the degree to which this hypothesis is consistent with the sample data which are summarized in the 2 × 2 contingency table.

3.2. Details of the Test

Consider a simple experiment which has only two possible outcomes, e.g., tumor presence or absence, graft rejection or acceptance, 6-month survival or death prior to that time. For convenience, we shall use the generic labels 'success' and 'failure' to describe the two outcomes. 'Success' might be tumor absence, graft acceptance or 6-month survival; then 'failure' represents tumor presence, graft rejection or death prior to 6 months, respectively. In each case, we can associate a rate or proportion with each of the categories success and failure; these will be numbers between 0 and 1 which have the property that their sum is always 1, since success and failure are the only possible outcomes. We could describe each rate or proportion equally well as the probability of the corresponding outcome, whether success or failure. Then if p represents the probability of success, the probability of failure will be $1-p$ since the probabilities of all possible outcomes in a population always sum to 1.

Table 3.1. A 2×2 table summarizing binary data collected from two groups

	Success	Failure	Total
Group 1	T	$R_1 - T$	R_1
Group 2	$C_1 - T$	$C_2 + T - R_1$	R_2
Total	C_1	C_2	N

In the basic model for the population, we assume that each individual has a probability of success which can be specified by a value of p between 0 and 1. Therefore, the aim of the study which is summarized in a 2×2 contingency table might be to compare two population groups, 1 and 2 say, with respect to their probabilities of success. To devise a test of significance suited to this purpose we must also assume:

(a) The probabilities of success for each member of Groups 1 and 2 are p_1 and p_2, respectively; i.e., within each group the probability of success does not vary from individual to individual.

(b) For any member of either group, the outcome which occurs (success/failure) does not influence the outcome for any other individual.

Once the data for the study have been collected (number of successes, failures in each group), they can be summarized in a 2×2 contingency table such as the one shown in Table 3.1.

The symbols R_1 and R_2 represent the total numbers of observations from Groups 1 and 2, respectively; the letter R is used because these are row totals for the table. Likewise, C_1 and C_2 represent the column totals for the categories Success and Failure. The total number of observations in the sample is N, and clearly $N = R_1 + R_2 = C_1 + C_2$. We will discuss the choice of letters appearing in the four cells of the 2×2 table shortly. First, however, we need to specify the null hypothesis for Fisher's test.

As we indicated above, it is quite natural in this particular situation to compare the probabilities of success in Groups 1 and 2. Therefore, the null hypothesis for Fisher's test may be expressed concisely as the statement H_0: $p_1 = p_2$, i.e., the probability of success is the same for Groups 1 and 2.

The letter T in the upper left corner of the contingency table shown in Table 3.1 represents the total number of successes observed in Group 1. The variable T is the test statistic for the observed data which we referred to in §2.3. Notice that since the numbers of individuals from Groups 1 and 2 are known (R_1 and R_2, respectively), as are the numbers of successes and failures

(C_1 and C_2, respectively), the remaining three entries in the table can be obtained by subtraction from row or column totals once the value of T has been determined. In effect, when the row and column totals are known, T determines the split of the successes between Groups 1 and 2; this is the principal reason that T is chosen as the test statistic for the significance test.

To determine the set of comparable events, we must consider all the possible 2×2 tables with row totals R_1, R_2 and column totals C_1, C_2 which might have been obtained. These can be identified by allowing the value of T to vary, beginning with the smallest possible value it can assume; this will usually be 0. Figure 3.1 displays four of these tables, provided both R_1 and C_1 are at least three and C_1 is at most R_2. As we saw in the example which was discussed in §2.2, these tables can be conveniently labelled using the value which the test statistic, T, assumes in the table. Clearly, the last table in the list will be one having a value of T which is equal to the smaller of R_1 and C_1.

To obtain the significance level of the test, we need the probability that, for known values of R_1, R_2 and C_1, the split of successes between Groups 1 and 2 is T and C_1-T, respectively. To calculate this probability, we must assume that the null hypothesis is true, i.e., that $p_1 = p_2$, and also that the sampling uncertainty is random. Certain fairly simple mathematical arguments lead to the formula

$$\frac{\binom{R_1}{t} \binom{N-R_1}{C_1-t}}{\binom{N}{C_1}}$$

for the probability that Table t, i.e., the 2×2 table with t successes in Group 1 and $C_1 - t$ in Group 2, would be observed if these assumptions are true. The symbols $\binom{R_1}{t}$, $\binom{N-R_1}{C_1-t}$ and $\binom{N}{C_1}$ used in this expression are called binomial coefficients. The binomial coefficient $\binom{n}{j}$ can be evaluated using the formula

$$\binom{n}{j} = \frac{n(n-1)(n-2)\ldots(n-j+2)(n-j+1)}{j(j-1)(j-2)\ldots(2)(1)}.$$

However, statistical tables are normally used to determine the significance level of Fisher's test. In any case, the most important aspect to remember is that the probability corresponding to each possible table, i.e., each value of the test statistic T, can be calculated.

Table 0

	Success	Failure	Total
Group 1	0	R_1	R_1
Group 2	C_1	R_2-C_1	R_2
Total	C_1	C_2	N

Table 1

	Success	Failure	Total
Group 1	1	R_1-1	R_1
Group 2	C_1-1	R_2-C_1+1	R_2
Total	C_1	C_2	N

Table 2

	Success	Failure	Total
Group 1	2	R_1-2	R_1
Group 2	C_1-2	R_2-C_1+2	R_2
Total	C_1	C_2	N

Table 3

	Success	Failure	Total
Group 1	3	R_1-3	R_1
Group 2	C_1-3	R_2-C_1+3	R_2
Total	C_1	C_2	N

Fig. 3.1. Four possible 2×2 tables having row totals R_1, R_2 and column totals C_1, C_2.

Once the numerical values of the probability distribution of T have been determined, there is a simple ranking for all the possible tables. This is based on the value of the probability corresponding to each table. If t_1 and t_2 are two possible values of T and the probability corresponding to Table t_1 is greater than the probability for Table t_2, then we say that Table t_1 is more consistent with the null hypothesis that $p_1 = p_2$ than Table t_2. On this basis we can quickly rank all the tables, i.e., all possible values of the test statistic T.

Table 3.2. The results of an experiment comparing the anti-tumor activity of two drugs in leukemic mice

	Complete remission		Total
	yes	no	
Methyl GAG	7	3	10
6-MP	2	7	9
Total	9	10	19

To complete the test, we must calculate the significance level of the data with respect to the null hypothesis. From the original 2×2 table which we observed and the corresponding value of T, we can determine the position of the observed 2×2 table in the ranking. Then, by summing the probabilities for possible tables whose rankings are no more consistent than the observed 2×2 table, we obtain the significance level of the data with respect to the null hypothesis that $p_1 = p_2$.

To illustrate each aspect of Fisher's test in a specific case, we consider the following example. Two drugs, methyl GAG and 6-MP, were screened in a small experiment to determine which, if either, demonstrated greater anti-tumor activity in leukemic mice. Ten mice received methyl GAG and nine were treated with 6-MP. When the experiment was ended, seven of the nine mice which had achieved complete remission belonged to the methyl GAG group. Table 3.2 summarizes the results of the experiment as a 2×2 contingency table.

In this particular case, mice in complete remission represent observed successes and the null hypothesis for this set of data states that $p_1 = p_2$, i.e., the probability of complete remission is the same for both drugs. The observed value of the test statistic, T, is seven, the number of complete remissions observed in mice treated with methyl GAG. Since nine, the total number of complete remissions observed, is the largest number that might have been obtained in the methyl GAG group, there are ten possible 2×2 tables, corresponding to the values of T from zero through nine. These tables are displayed in Figure 3.2, and the probability distribution for T is given in Table 3.3. From the probability distribution for T, we can determine the ranking of the ten possible tables. In this particular case it turns out that Table 5 is most consistent with the null hypothesis and Table 0 is the least

Table 0				Table 1			
	Complete remission		Total		Complete remission		Total
	yes	no			yes	no	
Methyl GAG	0	10	10		1	9	10
6-MP	9	0	9		8	1	9
Total	9	10	19		9	10	19

Table 2				Table 3			
Methyl GAG	2	8	10	3	7	10
6-MP	7	2	9	6	3	9
Total	9	10	19	9	10	19

Table 4				Table 5			
Methyl GAG	4	6	10	5	5	10
6-MP	5	4	9	4	5	9
Total	9	10	19	9	10	19

Table 6				Table 7			
Methyl GAG	6	4	10	7	3	10
6-MP	3	6	9	2	7	9
Total	9	10	19	9	10	19

Table 8				Table 9			
Methyl GAG	8	2	10	9	1	10
6-MP	1	8	9	0	9	9
Total	9	10	19	9	10	19

Fig. 3.2. The ten possible 2×2 tables having row totals 10, 9 and column totals, 9, 10.

Table 3.3. The probability of observing each of the tables shown in Figure 3.2 if the null hypothesis $H_0:p_1 = p_2$ is true

T (table #)	Probability	T (table #)	Probability
0	0.00001	5	0.3437
1	0.0009	6	0.1910
2	0.0175	7	0.0468
3	0.1091	8	0.0044
4	0.2864	9	0.00019

consistent of all 10. Notice that the observed result, Table 7, is fifth in the ranking, followed, in order, by Tables 2, 8, 1, 9 and 0. Therefore, since Tables 7, 2, 8, 1, 9 and 0 are each no more consistent with the null hypothesis than the observed result (Table 7), the significance level of the test is obtained by summing the probabilities for these six tables. The sum, 0.0698, is therefore the significance level of the data with respect to the null hypothesis that the probability of complete remission is the same for both drugs. And since the significance level is roughly 0.07, we conclude that there is no substantial evidence in the data to contradict the null hypothesis.

On the basis of this small experiment, we would conclude that the anti-tumor activity of methyl GAG and 6-MP in leukemic mice is apparently comparable, although further investigation might be justified.

3.3. Using Statistical Tables for Fisher's Test

As we indicated in the preceding section, the significance level for Fisher's test is usually determined by referring to specialized statistical tables (cf. Table 3.4). Since Table 3.4 is the first table of this kind that we have introduced, it is unfortunate that it is also the most complicated table which we will ask the reader to master. Nevertheless, to use Table 3.4, it is only necessary to arrange a 2×2 table of the data in standard form, i.e., the form assumed by the statistical tables. Figure 3.3 shows a 2×2 contingency table in standard form.

Table 3.4. Critical values for Fisher's test in 2×2 tables

R_1	R_2	C_1	0.05	0.025	0.01	0.001
4	4	4	0, 4			
	3	4	–, 4			
		3	0, –			
5	5	5	0, 5	0, 5	0, 5	
		4	0, 4			
	4	5	1, 5	–, 5	–, 5	
		4	0, 4	0, –	0, –	
		3	0, –			
	3	5	–, 5	–, 5		
		3	0, –	0, –		
	2	5	–, 5			
		2	0, –			
6	6	6	0, 6	0, 6	0, 6	
		5	0, 5	0, 5		
	5	6	1, 6	1, 6	–, 6	
		5	0, 5	0, 5	0, –	
		4	0, –	0, –		
	4	6	–, 6	–, 6	–, 6	
		5	1, 5			
		4	0, –	0, –	0, –	
		3	0, –			
	3	6	–, 6	–, 6		
		5	–, 5			
		4	1, –			
		3	0, –	0, –		
	2	6	–, 6			
		2	0, –			
7	7	7	1, 6	0, 7	0, 7	0, 7
		6	0, 6	0, 6	0, 6	
		5	0, 5	0, 5		
	6	7	1, 6	1, 7	1, 7	–, 7
		6	1, 6	0, 6	0, 6	0, –
		5	0, 5	0, 5	0, –	
		4	0, –	0, –		
	5	7	2, 7	–, 7	–, 7	
		6	1, 6	1, 6		
		5	0, 5	0, –	0, –	
		4	0, –	0, –		
		3	0, –			
	4	7	–, 7	–, 7	–, 7	
		6	–, 6	–, 6		
		5	1, –	1, –		
		4	0, –	0, –	0, –	
		3	0, –	0, –		
7	3	7	–, 7	–, 7	–, 7	
		6	–, 6			
		4	1, –			
		3	0, –	0, –	0, –	
	2	7	–, 7			
		2	0, –			
8	8	8	1, 7	1, 7	0, 8	0, 8
		7	1, 6	0, 7	0, 7	
		6	0, 6	0, 6	0, 6	
		5	0, 5			
	7	8	2, 7	1, 7	1, 8	–, 8
		7	1, 6	1, 7	0, 7	0, –
		6	1, 6	0, 6	0, 6	
		5	0, 5	0, –	0, –	
		4	0, –			
	6	8	2, 7	2, 8	2, 8	–, 8
		7	1, 7	1, 7	1, 7	
		6	1, 6	0, 6	0, 6	0, –
		5	0, 5	0, –	0, –	
		4	0, –	0, –		
	5	8	–, 7	–, 8	–, 8	–, 8
		7	2, 7	2, 7	–, 7	
		6	1, 6	1, 6	1, –	
		5	1, –	0, –	0, –	0, –
		4	0, –	0, –	0, –	
		3	0, –			
	4	8	–, 8	–, 8	–, 8	
		7	–, 7	–, 7		
		5	1, –	1, –		
		4	0, –	0, –	0, –	
		3	0, –	0, –		
	3	8	–, 8	–, 8	–, 8	
		7	–, 7	–, 7		
		4	1, –	1, –		
		3	0, –	0, –	0, –	
	2	8	–, 8	–, 8		
		2	0, –	0, –		
9	9	9	1, 8	1, 8	1, 8	0, 9
		8	1, 7	1, 7	0, 8	0, 8
		7	1, 6	0, 7	0, 7	
		6	0, 6	0, 6	0, 6	
		5	0, 5			

Table 3.4 (continued)

R_1	R_2	C_1	0.05	0.025	0.01	0.001	R_1	R_2	C_1	0.05	0.025	0.01	0.001
9	8	9	2, 8	2, 8	1, 8	1, 9	10	10	10	2, 8	2, 8	1, 9	0, 10
		8	1, 7	1, 7	1, 8	0, 8			9	1, 8	1, 8	1, 8	0, 9
		7	1, 6	1, 7	0, 7	0, –			8	1, 7	1, 7	0, 8	0, 8
		6	1, 6	0, 6	0, 6				7	0, 7	0, 7	0, 7	
		5	0, 5	0, –	0, –				6	0, 6	0, 6		
		4	0, –						5	0, 5			
	7	9	2, 8	2, 8	2, 8	–, 9		9	10	2, 8	2, 8	2, 9	1, 10
		8	2, 7	1, 8	1, 8				9	2, 8	2, 8	1, 8	0, 9
		7	1, 7	1, 7	1, 7	0, –			8	1, 7	1, 7	1, 8	0, 8
		6	1, 6	0, 6	0, –	0, –			7	1, 7	1, 7	0, 7	0, –
		5	0, 5	0, –	0, –				6	0, 6	0, 6	0, –	
		4	0, –	0, –					5	0, 5	0, –		
	6	9	3, 8	–, 8	–, 9	–, 9			4	0, –			
		8	2, 7	2, 8	2, 8			8	10	3, 9	3, 9	2, 9	–, 10
		7	2, 7	1, 7	1, 7				9	2, 8	2, 8	1, 9	1, 9
		6	1, 6	1, –	0, –	0, –			8	1, 7	1, 7	1, 8	0, –
		5	0, 5	0, –	0, –				7	1, 7	1, 7	0, 7	0, –
		4	0, –	0, –					6	1, 6	0, 6	0, –	
		3	0, –						5	0, 5	0, –	0, –	
	5	9	–, 8	–, 8	–, 9	–, 9			4	0, –	0, –		
		8	3, 8	–, 8	–, 8			7	10	3, 9	3, 9	3, 9	–, 10
		7	2, 7	2, 7					9	3, 8	2, 8	2, 9	–, 9
		6	1, 6	1, –	1, –				8	2, 7	2, 8	1, 8	1, –
		5	1, –	1, –	0, –	0, –			7	1, 7	1, 7	1, 7	0, –
		4	0, –	0, –	0, –				6	1, 6	1, –	0, –	0, –
		3	0, –						5	0, 5	0, –	0, –	
	4	9	–, 9	–, 9	–, 9				4	0, –	0, –		
		8	–, 8	–, 8	–, 8			6	10	4, 9	–, 9	–, 9	–, 10
		7	–, 7	–, 7					9	3, 8	3, 9	–, 9	–, 9
		6	2, –	2, –					8	2, 8	2, 8	2, 8	
		5	1, –	1, –	1, –				7	2, 7	1, 7	1, –	1, –
		4	0, –	0, –	0, –				6	1, 6	1, –	1, –	0, –
		3	0, –	0, –					5	1, –	0, –	0, –	
	3	9	–, 9	–, 9	–, 9				4	0, –	0, –	0, –	
		8	–, 8	–, 8					3	0, –			
		7	–, 7					5	10	–, 9	–, 9	–, 10	–, 10
		5	2, –						9	4, 9	–, 9	–, 9	
		4	1, –	1, –					8	3, 8	–, 8	–, 8	
		3	0, –	0, –	0, –				7	2, 7	2, –	2, –	
		2	0, –						6	1, 6	1, –	1, –	
	2	9	–, 9	–, 9					5	1, –	1, –	0, –	0, –
		2	0, –	0, –					4	0, –	0, –	0, –	
									3	0, –	0, –		

Table 3.4 (continued)

R₁	R₂	C₁	0.05	0.025	0.01	0.001
10	4	10	–, 9	–, 10	–, 10	–, 10
		9	–, 9	–, 9	–, 9	
		8	–, 8	–, 8		
		6	2, –	2, –		
		5	1, –	1, –	1, –	
		4	1, –	0, –	0, –	0, –
		3	0, –	0, –		
	3	10	–, 10	–, 10	–, 10	
		9	–, 9	–, 9		
		8	–, 8			
		5	2, –			
		4	1, –	1, –		
		3	0, –	0, –	0, –	
		2	0, –			
	2	10	–, 10	–, 10		
		9	–, 9			
		3	1, –			
		2	0, –	0, –		
11	11	11	2, 9	2, 9	2, 9	1, 10
		10	2, 8	1, 9	1, 9	0, 10
		9	1, 8	1, 8	1, 8	0, 9
		8	1, 7	1, 7	0, 8	
		7	0, 7	0, 7	0, 7	
		6	0, 6	0, 6		
		5	0, 5			
	10	11	3, 9	2, 9	2, 9	1, 10
		10	2, 8	2, 9	2, 9	1, 10
		9	2, 8	1, 8	1, 8	0, 9
		8	1, 7	1, 7	1, 8	0, –
		7	1, 7	1, 7	0, 7	
		6	0, 6	0, 6	0, –	
		5	0, 5	0, –		
		4	0, –			
	9	11	3, 9	3, 9	3, 10	2, 10
		10	2, 9	2, 9	2, 9	1, 10
		9	2, 8	2, 8	1, 8	1, 9
		8	1, 7	1, 8	1, 8	0, –
		7	1, 7	1, 7	0, 7	0, –
		6	1, 6	0, 6	0, –	
		5	0, 5	0, –	0, –	
		4	0, –			

R₁	R₂	C₁	0.05	0.025	0.01	0.001
11	8	11	3, 9	3, 9	3, 10	–, 11
		10	3, 9	3, 9	2, 9	2, 10
		9	2, 8	2, 8	2, 9	1, 9
		8	2, 8	2, 8	1, 8	0, –
		7	1, 7	1, 7	1, –	0, –
		6	1, 6	0, 6	0, –	
		5	0, 5	0, –	0, –	
		4	0, –	0, –		
	7	11	4, 9	4, 10	–, 10	–, 11
		10	3, 9	3, 9	3, 10	–, 10
		9	3, 8	2, 9	2, 9	
		8	2, 8	2, 8	1, 8	1, –
		7	2, 7	1, 7	1, –	0, –
		6	1, 6	1, –	0, –	0, –
		5	1, –	0, –	0, –	
		4	0, –	0, –		
		3	0, –			
	6	11	5, 10	–, 10	–, 10	–, 11
		10	4, 9	–, 9	–, 10	–, 10
		9	3, 8	3, 9	3, 9	
		8	3, 8	2, 8	2, 8	
		7	2, 7	2, –	1, –	1, –
		6	1, 6	1, –	1, –	0, –
		5	1, –	0, –	0, –	0, –
		4	0, –	0, –	0, –	
		3	0, –			
	5	11	–, 10	–, 10	–, 11	–, 11
		10	–, 9	–, 10	–, 10	
		9	4, 9	–, 9	–, 9	
		8	3, 8			
		7	2, 7	2, –	2, –	
		6	2, –	1, –	1, –	
		5	1, –	1, –	0, –	0, –
		4	0, –	0, –	0, –	
		3	0, –	0, –		
	4	11	–, 10	–, 11	–, 11	–, 11
		10	–, 10	–, 10	–, 10	
		9	–, 9	–, 9		
		8	–, 8			
		7	3, –			
		6	2, –	2, –		
		5	1, –	1, –	1, –	
		4	1, –	0, –	0, –	0, –
		3	0, –	0, –	0, –	

Table 3.4 (continued)

R₁	R₂	C₁	0.05	0.025	0.01	0.001	R₁	R₂	C₁	0.05	0.025	0.01	0.001
11	3	11	–, 11	–, 11	–, 11		12	8	12	4, 10	4, 10	4, 11	–, 11
		10	–, 10	–, 10					11	4, 10	3, 10	3, 10	–, 11
		9	–, 9						10	3, 9	3, 9	2, 10	2, 10
		5	2, –						9	2, 8	2, 9	2, 9	1, –
		4	1, –	1, –					8	2, 8	2, 8	1, 8	1, –
		3	0, –	0, –	0, –				7	1, 7	1, 7	1, –	0, –
		2	0, –						6	1, 6	1, –	0, –	0, –
	2	11	–, 11	–, 11					5	0, –	0, –	0, –	
		10	–, 10						4	0, –	0, –		
		3	1, –						3	0, –			
		2	0, –	0, –				7	12	5, 10	5, 11	–, 11	–, 12
12	12	12	3, 9	2, 10	2, 10	1, 11			11	4, 10	4, 10	–, 10	–, 11
		11	2, 9	2, 9	1, 10	1, 10			10	3, 9	3, 9	3, 10	–, 10
		10	2, 8	1, 9	1, 9	0, 10			9	3, 9	3, 9	2, 9	2, –
		9	1, 8	1, 8	1, 8	0, 9			8	2, 8	2, 8	2, –	1, –
		8	1, 7	0, 8	0, 8				7	2, 7	1, 7	1, –	0, –
		7	0, 7	0, 7	0, 7				6	1, 6	1, –	1, –	0, –
		6	0, 6	0, 6					5	1, –	0, –	0, –	
		5	0, 5						4	0, –	0, –	0, –	
	11	12	3, 9	3, 10	2,10	2, 11			3	0, –			
		11	3, 9	2, 9	2, 10	1, 10		6	12	–, 11	–, 11	–, 11	–, 12
		10	2, 8	2, 9	1, 9	1, 10			11	5, 10	–, 10	–, 11	–, 11
		9	2, 8	1, 8	1, 8	0, 9			10	4, 9	4, 10	–, 10	
		8	1, 7	1, 8	1, 8	0, –			9	3, 9	3, 9	3, 9	
		7	1, 7	0, 7	0, 7				8	3, 8	2, 8	2, –	
		6	0, 6	0, 6	0, –				7	2, 7	2, –	1, –	1, –
		5	0, 5	0, –					6	1, –	1, –	1, –	0, –
		4	0, –						5	1, –	1, –	0, –	0, –
	10	12	4, 10	3, 10	3, 10	2, 11			4	0, –	0, –	0, –	
		11	3, 9	2, 10	2, 10	1, 11			3	0, –	0, –		
		10	2, 8	2, 9	2, 9	1, 10		5	12	–, 11	–, 11	–, 11	–, 12
		9	2, 8	1, 8	1, 9	0, 9			11	–, 10	–, 11	–, 11	–, 11
		8	1, 7	1, 8	1, 8	0, –			10	5, 10	–, 10	–, 10	
		7	1, 7	1, 7	0, 7	0, –			9	4, 9	–, 9	–, 9	
		6	0, 6	0, 6	0, –				8	3, 8	3, –	3, –	
		5	0, 5	0, –	0, –				7	2, 7	2, –	2, –	
		4	0, –						6	2, –	1, –	1, –	1, –
	9	12	4, 10	4, 10	3, 10	–, 11			5	1, –	1, –	1, –	0, –
		11	3, 9	3, 10	3, 10	2, 11			4	0, –	0, –	0, –	
		10	3, 9	2, 9	2, 9	1, 10			3	0, –	0, –		
		9	2, 8	2, 8	2, 9	1, –		4	12	–, 11	–, 12	–, 12	–, 12
		8	2, 8	1, 8	1, 8	0, –			11	–, 11	–, 11	–, 11	
		7	1, 7	1, 7	0, 7	0, –			10	–, 10	–, 10	–, 10	
		6	1, 6	0, 6	0, –				9	–, 9	–, 9		
		5	0, 5	0, –	0, –								
		4	0, –	0, –									

Table 3.4 (continued)

R_1	R_2	C_1	0.05	0.025	0.01	0.001
12	4	7	3, –	3, –		
		6	2, –	2, –	2, –	
		5	1, –	1, –	1, –	
		4	1, –	0, –	0, –	0, –
		3	0, –	0, –	0, –	
		2	0, –			
	3	12	–, 12	–, 12	–, 12	
		11	–, 11	–, 11	–, 11	
		10	–, 10	–, 10		
		9	–, 9			
		6	3, –			
		5	2, –	2, –		
		4	1, –	1, –	1, –	
		3	0, –	0, –	0, –	
		2	0, –			
	2	12	–, 12	–, 12		
		11	–, 11			
		3	1, –			
		2	0, –	0, –		
13	13	13	3, 10	3, 10	2, 11	1, 12
		12	3, 9	2, 10	2, 10	1, 11
		11	2, 9	2, 9	1, 10	1, 10
		10	2, 8	1, 9	1, 9	0, 10
		9	1, 8	1, 8	0, 9	0, 9
		8	1, 7	0, 8	0, 8	
		7	0, 7	0, 7	0, 7	
		6	0, 6	0, 6		
		5	0, 5			
	12	13	4, 10	3, 10	3, 11	2, 12
		12	3, 9	3, 10	2, 10	1, 11
		11	3, 9	2, 9	2, 10	1, 10
		10	2, 8	2, 9	1, 9	1, 10
		9	2, 8	1, 8	1, 9	0, 9
		8	1, 7	1, 8	0, 8	0, –
		7	1, 7	0, 7	0, 7	
		6	0, 6	0, 6	0, –	
		5	0, 5	0, –		
		4	0, –			
	11	13	4, 10	4, 11	3, 11	2, 12
		12	3, 10	3, 10	2, 11	2, 11
		11	3, 9	2, 9	2, 10	1, 11
		10	2, 8	2, 9	1, 9	1, 10
		9	2, 8	1, 8	1, 9	0, 9
		8	1, 7	1, 8	1, 8	0, –

R_1	R_2	C_1	0.05	0.025	0.01	0.001
13	11	7	1, 7	1, 7	0, 7	0, –
		6	0, 6	0, 6	0, –	
		5	0, 5	0, –		
		4	0, –			
	10	13	4, 10	4, 11	4, 11	3, 12
		12	4, 10	3, 10	3, 11	2, 11
		11	3, 9	3, 10	2, 10	2, 11
		10	3, 9	2, 9	2, 9	1, 10
		9	2, 8	2, 9	1, 9	1, –
		8	2, 8	1, 8	1, 8	0, –
		7	1, 7	1, 7	0, 7	0, –
		6	0, 6	0, 6	0, –	
		5	0, 5	0, –	0, –	
		4	0, –	0, –		
	9	13	5, 11	4, 11	4, 11	–, 12
		12	4, 10	4, 11	3, 11	3, 12
		11	3, 10	3, 10	3, 10	2, 11
		10	2, 9	2, 9	2, 10	1, 10
		9	2, 8	2, 9	2, 9	1, –
		8	2, 8	1, 8	1, 8	0, –
		7	1, 7	1, 7	1, –	0, –
		6	1, 6	1, –	0, –	
		5	0, –	0, –	0, –	
		4	0, –	0, –		
	8	13	5, 11	5, 11	5, 12	–, 12
		12	4, 10	4, 11	4, 11	–, 12
		11	4, 10	4, 10	3, 10	–, 11
		10	3, 9	3, 9	3, 10	2, –
		9	3, 9	2, 9	2, 9	1, –
		8	2, 8	2, 8	1, 8	1, –
		7	1, 7	1, 7	1, –	0, –
		6	1, 6	1, –	0, –	0, –
		5	1, –	0, –	0, –	
		4	0, –	0, –		
		3	0, –			
	7	13	6, 11	–, 11	–, 12	–, 13
		12	5, 11	5, 11	–, 11	–, 12
		11	4, 10	4, 10	4, 11	–, 11
		10	3, 10	3, 10	3, 10	
		9	3, 9	3, 9	2, 9	2, –
		8	2, 8	2, 8	2, –	1, –
		7	2, 7	2, –	1, –	0, –
		6	1, –	1, –	1, –	0, –
		5	1, –	0, –	0, –	
		4	0, –	0, –	0, –	
		3	0, –			

Table 3.4 (continued)

R₁	R₂	C₁	0.05	0.025	0.01	0.001	R₁	R₂	C₁	0.05	0.025	0.01	0.001
13	6	13	-, 11	-, 12	-, 12	-, 13	14	14	14	3, 11	3, 11	3, 11	2, 12
		12	6, 11	-, 11	-, 11	-, 12			13	3, 10	3, 10	2, 11	1, 12
		11	5, 10	5, 11	-, 11				12	2, 10	2, 10	2, 10	1, 11
		10	4, 10	4, 10	-, 10				11	2, 9	2, 9	1, 10	0, 11
		9	3, 9	3, 9	3, -				10	2, 8	1, 9	1, 9	0, 10
		8	3, 8	2, 8	2, -				9	1, 8	1, 8	0, 9	0, 9
		7	2, 7	2, -	2, -	1, -			8	1, 7	0, 8	0, 8	
		6	2, -	1, -	1, -	0, -			7	0, 7	0, 7	0, 7	
		5	1, -	1, -	0, -	0, -			6	0, 6	0, 6		
		4	0, -	0, -	0, -				5	0, 5			
		3	0, -	0, -				13	14	4, 11	4, 11	3, 11	2, 12
	5	13	-, 12	-, 12	-, 12	-, 13			13	3, 10	3, 10	3, 11	2, 12
		12	-, 11	-, 11	-, 12	-, 12			12	3, 10	3, 10	2, 10	1, 11
		11	-, 10	-, 11	-, 11				11	2, 9	2, 9	2, 10	1, 11
		10	5, 10	-, 10	-, 10				10	2, 8	2, 9	1, 9	0, 10
		9	4, 9						9	2, 8	1, 8	1, 9	0, 9
		8	3, 8	3, -	3, -				8	1, 7	1, 8	0, 8	0, -
		7	3, -	2, -	2, -				7	1, 7	0, 7	0, 7	
		6	2, -	2, -	1, -	1, -			6	0, 6	0, 6	0, -	
		5	1, -	1, -	1, -	0, -			5	0, 5	0, -		
		4	1, -	0, -	0, -				4	0, -			
		3	0, -	0, -				12	14	4, 11	4, 11	4, 12	3, 13
	4	13	-, 12	-, 12	-, 13	-, 13			13	4, 10	3, 11	3, 11	2, 12
		12	-, 12	-, 12	-, 12				12	3, 10	3, 10	2, 10	1, 11
		11	-, 11	-, 11	-, 11				11	3, 9	2, 9	2, 10	1, 11
		10	-, 10	-, 10					10	2, 9	2, 9	1, 9	1, 10
		9	-, 9						9	2, 8	1, 8	1, 9	0, 9
		8	4, -						8	1, 7	1, 8	1, 8	0, -
		7	3, -	3, -					7	1, 7	0, 7	0, 7	
		6	2, -	2, -	2, -				6	0, 6	0, 6	0, -	
		5	1, -	1, -	1, -				5	0, 5	0, -		
		4	1, -	1, -	0, -	0, -			4	0, -			
		3	0, -	0, -	0, -			11	14	5, 11	4, 11	4, 12	3, 13
		2	0, -						13	4, 10	4, 11	3, 11	3, 12
	3	13	-, 13	-, 13	-, 13				12	4, 10	3, 10	3, 11	2, 11
		12	-, 12	-, 12	-, 12				11	3, 9	3, 10	2, 10	1, 11
		11	-, 11	-, 11					10	3, 9	2, 9	2, 10	1, 10
		10	-, 10						9	2, 8	2, 9	1, 9	0, -
		6	3, -						8	1, 7	1, 8	1, 8	0, -
		5	2, -	2, -					7	1, 7	1, 7	0, 7	0, -
		4	1, -	1, -	1, -				6	0, 6	0, 6	0, -	
		3	0, -	0, -	0, -				5	0, 5	0, -	0, -	
		2	0, -	0, -					4	0, -			
	2	13	-, 13	-, 13	-, 13								
		12	-, 12										
		3	1, -										
		2	0, -	0, -	0, -								

Table 3.4 (continued)

R_1	R_2	C_1	0.05	0.025	0.01	0.001
14	10	14	5, 11	5, 12	4, 12	4, 13
		13	5, 11	4, 11	4, 12	3, 12
		12	4, 10	3, 11	3, 11	2, 12
		11	3, 9	3, 10	2, 10	2, 11
		10	3, 9	2, 9	2, 10	1, 10
		9	2, 8	2, 9	1, 9	1, –
		8	2, 8	1, 8	1, 8	0, –
		7	1, 7	1, 7	1, –	0, –
		6	0, 6	0, 6	0, –	
		5	0, –	0, –	0, –	
		4	0, –	0, –		
	9	14	6, 12	5, 12	5, 12	–, 13
		13	5, 11	4, 11	4, 12	–, 12
		12	4, 10	4, 11	4, 11	3, 12
		11	4, 10	3, 10	3, 10	2, 11
		10	3, 9	3, 10	2, 10	2, –
		9	2, 8	2, 9	2, 9	1, –
		8	2, 8	2, 8	1, 8	0, –
		7	1, 7	1, 7	1, –	0, –
		6	1, 6	1, –	0, –	0, –
		5	0, –	0, –	0, –	
		4	0, –	0, –		
		3	0, –			
	8	14	6, 12	6, 12	–, 12	–, 13
		13	5, 11	5, 12	5, 12	–, 13
		12	5, 11	4, 11	4, 11	–, 12
		11	4, 10	4, 10	3, 11	
		10	3, 9	3, 10	3, 10	2, –
		9	3, 9	2, 9	2, 9	1, –
		8	2, 8	2, 8	2, –	1, –
		7	1, 7	1, 7	1, –	0, –
		6	1, –	1, –	0, –	0, –
		5	1, –	0, –	0, –	
		4	0, –	0, –	0, –	
		3	0, –			
	7	14	7, 12	–, 12	–, 13	–, 13
		13	6, 12	6, 12	–, 12	–, 13
		12	5, 11	5, 11	5, 12	–, 12
		11	4, 10	4, 10	4, 11	
		10	4, 10	4, 10	3, 10	
		9	3, 9	3, 9	2, 9	2, –
		8	2, 8	2, 8	2, –	1, –
		7	2, 7	2, –	1, –	1, –
		6	1, –	1, –	1, –	0, –
		5	1, –	0, –	0, –	
		4	0, –	0, –	0, –	
		3	0, –			

R_1	R_2	C_1	0.05	0.025	0.01	0.001
14	6	14	–, 12	–, 13	–, 13	–, 14
		13	–, 12	–, 12	–, 12	–, 13
		12	6, 11	–, 11	–, 12	–, 12
		11	5, 10	5, 11	–, 11	
		10	4, 10	4, 10		
		9	4, 9	3, 9	3, –	
		8	3, 8	3, –	2, –	2, –
		7	2, –	2, –	2, –	1, –
		6	2, –	1, –	1, –	0, –
		5	1, –	1, –	0, –	0, –
		4	0, –	0, –	0, –	
		3	0, –	0, –		
	5	14	–, 13	–, 13	–, 13	–, 14
		13	–, 12	–, 12	–, 13	–, 13
		12	–, 11	–, 12	–, 12	
		11	6, 11	–, 11	–, 11	
		10	5, 10	–, 10		
		9	4, 9	4, –		
		8	3, 8	3, –	3, –	
		7	3, –	2, –	2, –	
		6	2, –	2, –	1, –	1, –
		5	1, –	1, –	1, –	0, –
		4	1, –	0, –	0, –	
		3	0, –	0, –		
	4	14	–, 13	–, 13	–, 14	–, 14
		13	–, 12	–, 13	–, 13	
		12	–, 12	–, 12	–, 12	
		11	–, 11	–, 11		
		10	–, 10	–, 10		
		8	4, –	4, –		
		7	3, –	3, –		
		6	2, –	2, –	2, –	
		5	2, –	1, –	1, –	
		4	1, –	1, –	0, –	0, –
		3	0, –	0, –	0, –	
		2	0, –			
	3	14	–, 14	–, 14	–, 14	
		13	–, 13	–, 13	–, 13	
		12	–, 12	–, 12		
		11	–, 11			
		6	3, –			
		5	2, –	2, –		
		4	1, –	1, –	1, –	
		3	0, –	0, –	0, –	
		2	0, –	0, –		

Table 3.4 (continued)

R_1	R_2	C_1	0.05	0.025	0.01	0.001
14	2	14	–, 14	–, 14	–, 14	
		13	–, 13	–, 13		
		12	–, 12			
		4	2, –			
		3	1, –	1, –		
		2	0, –	0, –	0, –	
15	15	15	4, 11	3, 12	3, 12	2, 13
		14	3, 11	3, 11	3, 11	2, 12
		13	3, 10	2, 11	2, 11	1, 12
		12	2, 10	2, 10	2, 10	1, 11
		11	2, 9	2, 9	1, 10	0, 11
		10	1, 9	1, 9	1, 9	0, 10
		9	1, 8	1, 8	0, 9	0, 9
		8	1, 7	0, 8	0, 8	
		7	0, 7	0, 7	0, 7	
		6	0, 6	0, 6		
		5	0, 5			
	14	15	4, 11	4, 12	4, 12	3, 13
		14	4, 11	3, 11	3, 11	2, 12
		13	3, 10	3, 11	3, 11	2, 12
		12	3, 10	2, 10	2, 10	1, 11
		11	2, 9	2, 9	2, 10	1, 11
		10	2, 9	2, 9	1, 9	0, 10
		9	1, 8	1, 8	1, 9	0, 9
		8	1, 7	1, 8	0, 8	0, –
		7	1, 7	0, 7	0, 7	
		6	0, 6	0, 6	0, –	
		5	0, 5	0, –		
		4	0, –			
	13	15	5, 12	4, 12	4, 12	3, 13
		14	4, 11	4, 11	3, 12	2, 13
		13	3, 10	3, 11	3, 11	2, 12
		12	3, 10	3, 10	2, 10	1, 11
		11	2, 9	2, 9	2, 10	1, 11
		10	2, 9	2, 9	1, 9	0, 10
		9	2, 8	1, 8	1, 9	0, 9
		8	1, 7	1, 8	0, 8	0, –
		7	1, 7	0, 7	0, 7	
		6	0, 6	0, 6	0, –	
		5	0, 5	0, –		
		4	0, –			
	12	15	5, 12	5, 12	4, 12	3, 13
		14	4, 11	4, 11	4, 12	3, 13
		13	4, 11	4, 11	3, 11	2, 12

R_1	R_2	C_1	0.05	0.025	0.01	0.001
15	12	12	3, 10	3, 10	3, 11	2, 12
		11	3, 9	3, 10	2, 10	1, 11
		10	2, 9	2, 9	2, 10	1, 10
		9	2, 8	1, 8	1, 9	0, –
		8	1, 7	1, 8	1, 8	0, –
		7	1, 7	1, 7	0, 7	0, –
		6	0, 6	0, 6	0, –	
		5	0, 5	0, –	0, –	
		4	0, –			
	11	15	5, 12	5, 12	5, 13	4, 13
		14	5, 11	5, 12	4, 12	3, 13
		13	4, 11	4, 11	3, 12	3, 12
		12	4, 10	3, 10	3, 11	2, 12
		11	3, 10	3, 10	2, 10	2, 11
		10	3, 9	2, 9	2, 10	1, 10
		9	2, 8	2, 9	1, 9	1, –
		8	2, 8	1, 8	1, 8	0, –
		7	1, 7	1, 7	0, –	0, –
		6	0, 6	0, 6	0, –	
		5	0, –	0, –	0, –	
		4	0, –	0, –		
	10	15	6, 12	6, 13	5, 13	5, 14
		14	5, 11	5, 12	4, 12	4, 13
		13	5, 11	4, 11	4, 12	3, 12
		12	4, 10	4, 11	3, 11	3, 12
		11	4, 10	3, 10	3, 11	2, 11
		10	3, 9	2, 9	2, 10	1, 10
		9	2, 8	2, 9	2, 9	1, –
		8	2, 8	1, 8	1, 8	0, –
		7	1, 7	1, 7	1, –	0, –
		6	1, –	1, –	0, –	
		5	0, –	0, –	0, –	
		4	0, –	0, –		
	9	15	6, 12	6, 13	6, 13	–, 14
		14	6, 12	5, 12	5, 13	–, 13
		13	5, 11	5, 12	4, 12	4, 13
		12	4, 11	4, 11	4, 11	3, 12
		11	4, 10	3, 10	3, 11	2, 11
		10	3, 9	3, 10	2, 10	2, –
		9	3, 9	2, 9	2, 9	1, –
		8	2, 8	2, 8	1, 8	1, –
		7	1, 7	1, 7	1, –	0, –
		6	1, –	1, –	0, –	0, –
		5	1, –	0, –	0, –	
		4	0, –	0, –		
		3	0, –			

Table 3.4 (continued)

R_1	R_2	C_1	0.05	0.025	0.01	0.001
15	8	15	7, 13	7, 13	–, 13	–, 14
		14	6, 12	6, 12	6, 13	–, 14
		13	5, 11	5, 12	5, 12	–, 13
		12	5, 11	4, 11	4, 11	–, 12
		11	4, 10	4, 11	4, 11	3, –
		10	4, 10	3, 10	3, 10	2, –
		9	3, 9	3, 9	2, 9	1, –
		8	2, 8	2, 8	2, –	1, –
		7	2, –	1, –	1, –	0, –
		6	1, –	1, –	1, –	0, –
		5	1, –	0, –	0, –	
		4	0, –	0, –	0, –	
		3	0, –			
	7	15	–, 13	–, 13	–, 14	–, 14
		14	7, 13	7, 13	–, 13	–, 14
		13	6, 12	6, 12	–, 12	–, 13
		12	5, 11	5, 11	5, 12	–, 12
		11	4, 11	4, 11	4, 11	
		10	4, 10	4, 10	3, 10	3, –
		9	3, 9	3, 9	3, –	2, –
		8	2, 8	2, 8	2, –	1, –
		7	2, –	2, –	1, –	1, –
		6	1, –	1, –	1, –	0, –
		5	1, –	1, –	0, –	0, –
		4	0, –	0, –	0, –	
		3	0, –	0, –		
	6	15	–, 13	–, 14	–, 14	–, 15
		14	–, 13	–, 13	–, 13	–, 14
		13	7, 12	–, 12	–, 13	–, 13
		12	6, 11	6, 12	–, 12	
		11	5, 11	5, 11	–, 11	
		10	4, 10	4, 10	4, –	
		9	4, 9	3, 9	3, –	
		8	3, 8	3, –	2, –	2, –
		7	2, –	2, –	2, –	1, –
		6	2, –	1, –	1, –	0, –
		5	1, –	1, –	0, –	0, –
		4	0, –	0, –	0, –	
		3	0, –	0, –		
	5	15	–, 14	–, 14	–, 14	–, 15
		14	–, 13	–, 13	–, 14	–, 14
		13	–, 12	–, 13	–, 13	

R_1	R_2	C_1	0.05	0.025	0.01	0.001
15	5	12	–, 12	–, 12	–, 12	
		11	6, 11	–, 11	–, 11	
		10	5, 10			
		9	4, 9	–, 4	–, 4	
		8	3, –	3, –	3, –	
		7	3, –	2, –	2, –	
		6	2, –	2, –	1, –	1, –
		5	1, –	1, –	1, –	0, –
		4	1, –	0, –	0, –	
		3	0, –	0, –	0, –	
	4	15	–, 14	–, 14	–, 15	–, 15
		14	–, 13	–, 14	–, 14	
		13	–, 13	–, 13	–, 13	
		12	–, 12	–, 12	–, 12	
		11	–, 11	–, 11		
		10	–, 10			
		9	5, –			
		8	4, –	4, –		
		7	3, –	3, –	3, –	
		6	2, –	2, –	2, –	
		5	2, –	1, –	1, –	
		4	1, –	1, –	0, –	0, –
		3	0, –	0, –	0, –	
		2	0, –			
	3	15	–, 15	–, 15	–, 15	
		14	–, 14	–, 14	–, 14	
		13	–, 13	–, 13		
		12	–, 12	–, 12		
		11	–, 11			
		7	4, –			
		6	3, –	3, –		
		5	2, –	2, –		
		4	1, –	1, –	1, –	
		3	0, –	0, –	0, –	
		2	0, –	0, –		
	2	15	–, 15	–, 15	–, 15	
		14	–, 14	–, 14		
		13	–, 13			
		4	2, –			
		3	1, –	1, –		
		2	0, –	0, –	0, –	

	Success	Failure	Total
Group 1	T	$R_1 - T$	R_1
Group 2	$C_1 - T$	$C_2 - R_1 + T$	R_2
Total	C_1	C_2	N

$R_1 \geqslant R_2$ and $C_1 \leqslant C_2$.

Fig. 3.3. A 2×2 contingency table in standard form.

To eliminate unnecessary tabulation in preparing statistical tables for Fisher's test, we have adopted the convention that $R_1 \geqslant R_2$ and $C_1 \leqslant C_2$. Thus, in standard form, the larger sample is designated as Group 1, while the generic label 'Success' corresponds to the binary category with the smaller number of observed outcomes. With Groups 1 and 2 and the categories Success and Failure thus determined, the 2×2 table is now in standard form.

To use Table 3.4 for determining the significance level of Fisher's test, first identify the values of R_1, R_2 and C_1 from the 2×2 table in standard form. Next, locate the row in Table 3.4 corresponding to these values of R_1, R_2 and C_1. Notice that in the columns labelled 0.05, 0.025, 0.01 and 0.001, pairs of numbers are tabulated; these are called the 0.05, 0.025, 0.01 and 0.001 critical values, respectively. Let n_L represent the left-hand or lower critical value in the 0.05 column, say, and n_U represent the right-hand or upper 0.05 critical value. If t_o is the observed value of T in the 2×2 table (see Figure 3.3 for the location of T) and if $t_o \leqslant n_L$ *or* $t_o \geqslant n_u$, the significance level of the data with respect to the null hypothesis is at most 0.05, i.e., $p \leqslant 0.05$. When only n_L is tabulated in the 0.05 column, then the significance level of the data is at most 0.05 provided $t_o \leqslant n_L$; there is no possible observed value of T greater than n_L such that $p \leqslant 0.05$. Similarly, if only n_U appears in the 0.05 column, then $p \leqslant 0.05$ provided $t_o \geqslant n_U$; there is no possible observed value of T less than n_U such that $p \leqslant 0.05$. Finally, if neither n_L nor n_U is tabulated, there is no possible observed value of T, for the given combination of R_1, R_2 and C_1, such that the significance level of the data is at most 0.05.

By using the pairs of critical values for 0.025, 0.01 and 0.001 in exactly the same way, we can obtain corresponding bounds on the significance level of Fisher's test, i.e., $p \leq 0.025$, $p \leq 0.01$ and $p \leq 0.001$, respectively. Of course, if the significance level of the data exceeds 0.05, i.e., if $n_L < t_o < n_U$, it is pointless to check the other critical values, since we already know that $p > 0.05$.

To illustrate the use of Table 3.4, we return to the example discussed in §3.2 involving 19 leukemic mice treated with methyl GAG or 6-MP. The 2×2 table for this example is given in Table 3.2. The methyl GAG sample is larger than the 6-MP sample; therefore, the rows of Table 3.2 are in standard form. And since the nine mice in complete remission is a smaller number than the remaining ten, it follows that Table 3.2 is already in standard form. Thus, $R_1 = 10$, $R_2 = 9$, $C_1 = 9$ and the observed value of T is $t_o = 7$. We now refer to the appropriate row of Table 3.4. The 0.05 critical values are 2 and 8. Since $2 < t_o = 7 < 8$, it follows that, in this case, the observed value of T lies between n_L and n_U. Therefore, the significance level of this data with respect to the null hypothesis exceeds 0.05, i.e., $p > 0.05$. In fact, in §3.2 we calculated that $p = 0.07$. The use of Table 3.4 makes it easy to apply Fisher's test to a given set of data; however, if the significance level must be known exactly, it will usually be necessary to ask a statistician to do the calculations discussed in §3.2.

The following example, which involves rearranging a 2×2 table to put it in standard form, illustrates the situation which is usually encountered in applying Fisher's test to a particular set of data.

As part of an experiment to investigate the value of infusing stored, autologous bone marrow as a means of restoring marrow function, a researcher administered Myleran to 15 dogs. Nine were then randomized to the treatment group and received an infusion of bone marrow, while the remaining six dogs served as a control group. The experiment was ended after 30 days and the results are presented in Table 3.5a.

To test the hypothesis that the probability of 30-day survival is the same in both groups of dogs, i.e., no treatment effect, we first need to put the 2×2 table in standard form. Since the treatment sample is larger, we designate the infused dogs (Treatment) as Group 1. The smaller number of observed outcomes corresponds to the five dogs that died prior to 30 days; therefore, we label this category Success. Table 3.5b shows the 2×2 table for the same experiment in standard form; clearly, $R_1 = 9$, $R_2 = 6$ and $C_1 = 5$. From the appropriate row of Table 3.4 we determine that since the observed value of T is 0 (see Table 3.5b), the significance level of the data is at most 0.01; more-

Table 3.5. Treatment and survival data for 15 dogs insulted with Myleran: (a) initial tabulation; (b) tabulated in standard form

a Initial tabulation

Bone marrow infusion	30-day survival		Total
	yes	no	
No (Control)	1	5	6
Yes (Treatment)	9	0	9
Total	10	5	15

b Tabulation in standard form

Bone marrow infusion	30-day survival		Total
	no (success)	yes (failure)	
Treatment (Group 1)	0	9	9
Control (Group 2)	5	1	6
Total	5	10	15

over, since there are no 0.001 critical values when $R_1 = 9$, $R_2 = 6$ and $C_1 = 5$, it follows that $p > 0.001$. Thus, the significance level of the data is between 0.01 and 0.001, i.e., $0.001 < p < 0.01$, and we conclude that the probability of 30-day survival is significantly higher in dogs which receive an infusion of stored, autologous bone marrow.

A few specialized books contain more extensive tables for applying Fisher's test than Table 3.4. However, few tables extend to situations where the larger row total exceeds 20. For these cases, there is an approximate version of Fisher's test which is usually adequate. Therefore, in chapter 4, we intend to describe in detail the approximate test for contingency tables.

4 Approximate Significance Tests for Contingency Tables

4.1. Introduction

Fisher's test, which we discussed in chapter 3, evaluates the exact significance level of the null hypothesis that the probability of success is the same in two distinct groups. Ideally, the exact significance level of this test is what we would prefer to calculate in every situation. However, the calculations are often rather formidable unless the contingency table is based on a small number of observations, and extensive statistical tables which cover all possible cases simply are not available; such tables would be too unwieldy and far too expensive. In situations like this, statisticians have frequently arranged to bypass formidable calculations, or the need for unwieldy sets of tables, by developing accurate approximations to particular tests. The approximate version of Fisher's test which we discuss in the following section is known as the χ^2 (chi-squared) test for 2×2 tables.

4.2. The χ^2 Test for 2×2 Tables

Suppose that a 2×2 table, such as the one shown in Table 4.1, has row and column totals which are too large for published statistical tables to be used in determining the significance level of Fisher's test. For reasons of convenience in describing the χ^2 test, we have chosen to label the entries in the 2×2 table O_{11}, O_{12}, O_{21} and O_{22} (see Table 4.1). The symbol O_{11} represents the observed number of successes in Group 1. If we call 'success' category I and 'failure' category II, then O_{11} is the number of category I observations in Group 1. Similarly, the symbol O_{12} is the number of category II observations (failures) in Group 1; the symbols O_{21} and O_{22} represent the corresponding category I (success) and category II (failure) totals for Group 2.

The assumptions on which the χ^2 test is based are the same as those for Fisher's test. If p_1 and p_2 represent the probabilities of category I for Groups 1 and 2, respectively, then we are assuming that:

(a) within each group the probability of category I (success) does not vary from individual to individual,

(b) for any member of the population, the outcome which occurs (I or II) does not influence the outcome for any other individual.

Likewise, the purpose of the χ^2 test is the same as that of Fisher's test, namely, to determine the degree to which the observed data are consistent with the null hypothesis H_0: $p_1 = p_2$, i.e., the probability of category I in the two groups is the same.

The basis for the χ^2 test is essentially this: assume that the null hypothesis, H_0, is true and caculate the 2×2 table which would be expected to occur based on this assumption and the row and column totals R_1, R_2, C_1 and C_2. If the observed 2×2 table is similar to the expected 2×2 table, the significance level of the data with respect to H_0 will be fairly large, say 0.5. However, if the observed 2×2 table is very different from the expected 2×2 table, the significance level of the data with respect to H_0 will be rather small, say 0.05 or less. In both cases, the approximation to Fisher's test occurs in the calculation of the significance level. And this is precisely the point at which the calculations for Fisher's test become so formidable when R_1, R_2, C_1 and C_2 are quite large.

In order to illustrate the calculations which the χ^2 test involves, we will consider the sample 2×2 table shown in Table 4.2. The data are taken from *Storb* et al. [1977] and summarize the outcomes of 68 bone marrow transplants for patients with aplastic anemia. Each patient was classified according to the outcome of the graft (Rejection, Yes or No) and also according to the size of the marrow cell dose which was used in the transplant procedure. The principal question which the data are intended to answer is whether the size of the marrow cell dose is associated with the marrow graft rejection rate.

To carry out the approximate test of significance, we need to calculate the values which would be expected in this particular sample if the null hypothesis, H_0, is true. This table of expected values will have the same row and column totals as the observed 2×2 table. In the 2×2 table shown in Table 4.3, the four entries are represented by the symbols e_{11}, e_{12}, e_{21} and e_{22} to distinguish them from the values in the observed 2×2 table (cf. Table 4.1). The meaning of the subscripts on these symbols should be fairly obvious. The symbol e_{11} represents the expected number of category I outcomes in Group 1, while e_{21} is the corresponding expected value for Group 2; likewise, e_{12} and e_{22} are the category II expected numbers for Groups 1 and 2, respectively.

Table 4.1. A 2×2 table summarizing binary data collected from two groups

	Success (I)	Failure (II)	Total
Group 1	O_{11}	O_{12}	R_1
Group 2	O_{21}	O_{22}	R_2
Total	C_1	C_2	N

Table 4.2. Graft rejection status and marrow cell dose data for 68 aplastic anemia patients

Graft rejection	Marrow cell dose (10^8 cells/kg)		Total
	< 3.0	$\geqslant 3.0$	
Yes	17	4	21
No	19	28	47
Total	36	32	68

Table 4.3. The 2×2 table of expected values corresponding to the observed data summarized in Table 4.1

	Success (I)	Failure (II)	Total
Group 1	e_{11}	e_{12}	R_1
Group 2	e_{21}	e_{22}	R_2
Total	C_1	C_2	N

The overall success rate in the observed 2×2 table is C_1/N. If the null hypothesis is true, this rate is a natural estimate of the common success rate for both Group 1 and Group 2. There are R_1 individuals in Group 1; therefore, if the null hypothesis is true, the expected number of category I outcomes (success) in Group 1 would be

$$e_{11} = R_1 \times \left(\frac{C_1}{N}\right) = \frac{R_1 \times C_1}{N}.$$

Notice that this is the product of the row total for Group 1 (R_1) and the column total for category I (C_1) divided by the total number of observations (N). This makes the formula particularly easy to recall and use. The other expected values in the 2×2 table are calculated from similar formulae, viz.

$$e_{12} = \frac{R_1 \times C_2}{N}, \quad e_{21} = \frac{R_2 \times C_1}{N} \quad \text{and } e_{22} = \frac{R_2 \times C_2}{N}.$$

Of course, since the row and column totals for the 2×2 table of expected numbers are already fixed (R_1, R_2, C_1 and C_2), we know from the discussion of Fisher's test (see § 3.2) that, once we have calculated e_{11}, we can obtain the other entries in the table of expected numbers by subtraction. One possible set of formulae for obtaining e_{12}, e_{21} and e_{22} in this way is

$$e_{12} = R_1 - e_{11}, \quad e_{21} = C_1 - e_{11} \quad \text{and } e_{22} = R_2 - e_{21}.$$

Although we could list other sets of formulae for calculating e_{12}, e_{21} and e_{22}, these versions will suffice. Any correct set will always produce a table of expected numbers having row and column totals R_1, R_2, C_1 and C_2. Remember that these expected values are based on the assumption that the null hypothesis, H_0, is true, i.e., the probability of category I (success) is the same for Groups 1 and 2. Table 4.4 shows the table of expected values for the data concerning bone marrow transplantation, including details of the calculations.

In § 2.3 we specified that an appropriate test statistic, T, is needed to carry out a test of significance. In the case of Fisher's test, T is the number of successes (category I) observed in Group 1. The choice of T, the test statistic, lies at the heart of the χ^2 approximation to Fisher's test. One formula for T is the expression

$$T = \frac{(O_{11} - e_{11})^2}{e_{11}} + \frac{(O_{12} - e_{12})^2}{e_{12}} + \frac{(O_{21} - e_{21})^2}{e_{21}} + \frac{(O_{22} - e_{22})^2}{e_{22}} = \sum_{i=1}^{2} \sum_{j=1}^{2} \frac{(O_{ij} - e_{ij})^2}{e_{ij}}.$$

We can see here that use of the summation symbol, Σ, which we introduced in chapter 1, greatly facilitates writing the formula for T. The use of two Σ symbols simply means that, in the expression $(O_{ij} - e_{ij})^2 / e_{ij}$, i is replaced by 1 and 2 and for each of these values j is replaced by 1 and 2. Thus, each of the four terms which must be summed is generated.

A slightly lengthier formula, involving an adjustment called Yates' continuity correction, specifies that

$$T = \sum_{i=1}^{2} \sum_{j=1}^{2} \frac{(|O_{ij} - e_{ij}| - \frac{1}{2})^2}{e_{ij}}.$$

The symbol $|\ldots|$ is mathematical shorthand which means 'use the non-negative value of the quantity between the vertical lines'. The continuity correc-

Table 4.4. The 2×2 table of expected values corresponding to the graft rejection data summarized in Table 4.2

Graft rejection	Marrow cell dose (10^8 cells/kg)		Total
	< 3.0	$\geqslant 3.0$	
Yes	$\dfrac{21 \times 36}{68} = 11.12$	$\dfrac{21 \times 32}{68} = 9.88$ $= 21 - 11.12$	21
No	$\dfrac{47 \times 36}{68} = 24.88$ $= 36 - 11.12$	$\dfrac{47 \times 32}{68} = 22.12$ $= 47 - 24.88$	47
Total	36	32	68

tion is obtained by subtracting ½ from each of the non-negative differences; this adjustment improves the probability approximation which we will discuss later. In order to calculate the value of T for a given sample of data, we must first obtain the 2×2 table of expected numbers and then use O_{11}, O_{12}, O_{21}, O_{22} and e_{11}, e_{12}, e_{21} and e_{22} in the formula. However, even this calculation can be reduced. Recall that the formulae for the entries in the table of expected numbers only use R_1, R_2, C_1, C_2 and N. If we replace e_{11}, e_{12}, e_{21} and e_{22} in the formula for T by their values in terms of row and column totals, it is possible to show that there is another formula for T which always gives the same value as the lengthy formula specified above. This alternative formula for T is

$$T = \frac{N(|O_{11}O_{22} - O_{12}O_{21}| - \tfrac{1}{2}N)^2}{R_1 R_2 C_1 C_2}.$$

Apart from the fact that this latter formula for T is more concise and involves less calculation, we notice at once that the shorter version does not require any of the values e_{11}, e_{12}, e_{21} or e_{22} from the 2×2 table of expected numbers. Therefore, by using the shorter formula, we avoid having to calculate these values at an intermediate step; nonetheless, the two formulae are exactly equivalent. If we use the data given in Table 4.2 to calculate T, the observed value of the test statistic is

$$\frac{68(|17 \times 28 - 4 \times 19| - 34)^2}{21 \times 47 \times 36 \times 32} = 8.01.$$

Though we certainly recommend use of the concise formula for T, there is an advantage in our having introduced the longer version first. For a given set of row and column totals (R_1, R_2, C_1 and C_2), the test statistic T could take on many different values, depending on the observed values O_{11}, O_{12}, O_{21} and O_{22}. Whatever this set of possible values of T might be, there are some common features which we can deduce by examining the longer formula for T. To begin with, each of the four terms in the long version of T must be positive; therefore, T will always be positive. Secondly, if each observed value, O_{ij}, is very close to its corresponding expected number, e_{ij}, then T will be very close to 0. Thus, a small value of T suggests that the observed data are consistent with the null hypothesis, i.e., the probability of category I (success) is the same for Groups 1 and 2. Conversely, if each O_{ij} is very different from the corresponding e_{ij}, then T should be rather large. Thus, a large value of T suggests that the observed data are not consistent with the null hypothesis. And so we see that if the observed value of T, for a particular set of data, is the number t_0 (for example, 8.01), then values of T which exceed t_0 correspond to possible 2×2 tables which are less consistent with the null hypothesis, H_0, than the 2×2 table which actually was observed ($T = t_0$). In order to calculate the significance level of the data, we simply need to sum the probabilities associated with all possible values of T which are greater than or equal to the observed value t_0, i.e., calculate $Pr(T \geq t_0)$. In the bone marrow transplant example this is precisely $Pr(T \geq 8.01)$.

As we indicated earlier, the heart of the χ^2 approximation to Fisher's test lies in the choice of the test statistic, T. We have already learned that 2×2 tables which are no more consistent with the null hypothesis than the observed 2×2 table ($T = t_0$) correspond to the set described by the inequality $T \geq t_0$. To obtain the probability of this set, we require the probability distribution of T when H_0 is true. And herein lies the importance of the choice of T as a test statistic. By means of complex mathematical arguments, statisticians have proved that when H_0 is true, i.e., when the probability of category I is the same in Groups 1 and 2, the test statistic T has a distribution which is approximately the same as the probability distribution called χ_1^2 (chi-squared with one degree of freedom). Therefore, we can determine the significance level of the data (recall that this is $Pr(T \geq t_0)$) by calculating the probability that $\chi_1^2 \geq t_0$. The shorthand notation $Pr(\chi_1^2 \geq t_0)$ represents the probability that a random variable, whose probability distribution is χ_1^2, exceeds t_0. Of course, this means that the significance level we calculate will be approximate; however, a great deal of statistical research has been devoted to showing that the approximation is quite accurate for most cases not covered by tables for Fisher's test.

To evaluate $Pr(\chi^2_1 \geq t_o)$ we must refer to statistical tables of the χ^2_1 distribution. In §4.3 we intend to introduce other members of the χ^2 family of probability distributions. For this reason, we have chosen to discuss the use of statistical tables for χ^2 probability distributions in the final section of this chapter. For our present purposes, it suffices to indicate that $Pr(\chi^2_1 \geq t_o)$ can be evaluated by referring to statistical tables. Therefore, the approximate significance level of the data with respect to the null hypothesis, H_0, can be determined.

To conclude the bone marrow transplant example we need to evaluate $Pr(\chi^2_1 \geq 8.01)$, since 8.01 is the observed value of T in this case. From tables for the χ^2_1 distribution we learn that $0.001 < Pr(\chi^2_1 \geq 8.01) < 0.005$. Since the exact value of $Pr(\chi^2_1 \geq 8.01)$ is still an approximate significance level, even if the approximation is quite accurate, the range $0.001-0.005$ is enough to indicate to us that the data represent very strong evidence against the null hypothesis that the graft rejection rate is the same for patients receiving the two different marrow cell doses. Not only does the graft rejection rate appear to be much smaller (4/32 versus 17/36) for patients transplanted with the larger dose, but on the basis of the χ^2 test we can state that this apparent difference is statistically significant, since the significance level of the test is $p < 0.005$.

Comments:

(a) Depending on experimental conditions, the observed results in a 2×2 table may be obtained from two essentially different experimental designs:

i.   The row totals R_1, R_2 are fixed by the experimenter in advance. For example, to compare 6-month survival rates under two chemotherapies, we might select 100 patients and randomize a predetermined number, say R_1, and the remainder, $100 - R_1$ (which therefore equals R_2), to the two treatment arms. Or, to compare the probability of tumor development after insult with croton oil in male and female mice, we would randomly select a fixed number of each sex. In this latter case we might have $R_1 = R_2 = 25$.

ii.   The row totals R_1, R_2 are random (not fixed in advance by the experimenter). This type of design would probably be used to compare marrow graft rejection rates among patients with and without prior transfusions, since the number of patients in these latter two categories usually cannot be fixed in advance. This design might also be used to compare the probability of tumor presence in adult mice which are dominant and recessive in some genetic characteristic.

Regardless of the experimental design, the null hypothesis on which the significance test is based remains unchanged, namely H_0: $p_1 = p_2$, i.e., the probability of category I (success) is the same for both groups.

(b) As we mentioned earlier, the distribution of the test statistic T is only approximately χ_1^2. In general, the accuracy of this approximation depends on the total numbers of observations in the rows and columns of the 2×2 table. A conservative rule-of-thumb for ensuring that the approximation is accurate requires that all the expected numbers, e_{ij}, exceed five. A more liberal rule allows one expected number to be as low as two. If the values in the 2×2 table of expected numbers are small, then Fisher's test should be used to evaluate the significance level of the data with respect to H_0.

4.3. The χ^2 Test for Rectangular Contingency Tables

In the preceding section, we considered the problem of analyzing binary data (i.e., Success/Failure, Response/No Response) collected from independent samples drawn from two populations (i.e., Control, Treatment). However, the simplicity of the 2×2 table is also a major disadvantage if initial tabulations of the observed data are more extensive than the binary categories Success and Failure. Clearly, reducing more detailed observations to simple binary categories results in lost information. The rectangular contingency table with, say, a rows and b columns generalizes the simple 2×2 table.

The basic model for the rectangular contingency table assumes that the outcome for each of N experimental units (patients, animals, lab tests, etc.) may be classified according to two schemes, A and B, say. If the classification categories for scheme A are labelled $A_1, A_2, \ldots, A_a$, then the observation for each member of a sample belongs to exactly one of these categories. For example, in a clinical trial design to compare the effects of PAS and streptomycin in the treatment of tuberculosis, each participant in the trial would be treated with one of PAS or streptomycin, or perhaps a combination of both drugs. In this case, A_1 might represent the PAS-only group, A_2 the streptomycin-only group and A_3 the combined drugs group. Similarly, if the classification categories under scheme B are labelled $B_1, B_2, \ldots, B_b$, then the outcome for each member of the sample belongs to exactly one of these categories as well. In the pulmonary tuberculosis clinical trial mentioned above, the

Table 4.5. A rectangular contingency table with a rows and b columns

Classification scheme A	Classification scheme B					Total
	B_1	B_2	$\cdot$	$\cdot$	$\cdot$	B_b	
A_1	O_{11}	O_{12}	$\cdot$	$\cdot$	$\cdot$	O_{1b}	R_1
A_2	O_{21}	O_{22}	$\cdot$	$\cdot$	$\cdot$	O_{2b}	R_2
$\cdot$			$\cdot$	$\cdot$		$\cdot$	$\cdot$
$\cdot$			$\cdot$	$\cdot$		$\cdot$	$\cdot$
$\cdot$			$\cdot$	$\cdot$		$\cdot$	$\cdot$
A_a	O_{a1}	O_{a2}	$\cdot$	$\cdot$	$\cdot$	O_{ab}	R_a
Total	C_1	C_2	$\cdot$	$\cdot$	$\cdot$	C_b	N

response of each patient to treatment, as measured by the analysis of a sputum sample, would be one of positive smear, negative smear and positive culture or negative smear and negative culture. In this case, we might label the patients having a positive smear B_1, those having a negative smear but positive culture B_2, and those with a negative smear and negative culture B_3.

The results of classifying each sample unit according to both schemes, A and B, may be concisely summarized in the rectangular contingency table shown in Table 4.5. In this $a \times b$ contingency table with a rows and b columns, each cell corresponds to a unique row and column combination. Therefore, each cell identifies the number of sample members which were classified as belonging to a unique, combined category of Scheme A *and* Scheme B. Paralleling our approach to 2×2 tables in §4.2, we have chosen to represent by O_{11} the number of sample members which are both A_1 and B_1. Similarly, the symbol O_{ij} denotes the total number of sample members which are both A_i and B_j. For example, the Medical Research Council [1950] reported the details of a clinical trial in which 273 patients were treated for pulmonary tuberculosis with one of PAS, streptomycin or a combination of the two drugs. A 3×3 cross-tabulation of the results of that trial is presented in Table 4.6.

In general, the null hypothesis which is tested using the χ^2 test for a rectangular contingency table is H_0: the A and B classification schemes are independent. Typically, this statement is interpreted in medical situations to mean that there is no association between the two classification schemes, A and B. For example, in the clinical trial involving the treatment of pulmonary tuberculosis with PAS, streptomycin or a combination of these two drugs, the

Table 4.6. Sputum analysis and treatment data for 273 pulmonary tuberculosis patients

Treatment	Sputum analysis			Total
	positive smear	negative smear, positive culture	negative smear, negative culture	
PAS only	56	30	13	99
Streptomycin only	46	18	20	84
Combined drugs	37	18	35	90
Total	139	66	68	273

null hypothesis of independence means that a patient's condition at the conclusion of the trial did not depend on the treatment received.

However, there is another null hypothesis which is tested in exactly the same way, and which may occasionally be more appropriate. If one of the classification schemes, say A, corresponds to sampling from a different groups, then H_0 can also be interpreted as specifying that the probability distribution of the B classification scheme is identical in all of the a groups. This is simply a generalization of the null hypothesis which we discussed in §4.2 in connection with the χ^2 test in 2×2 contingency tables. For example, suppose that the categories of scheme A represent three strains of mice, and the categories of B describe three types of tumors which are observed in a sample of 75 mice, 25 of each strain, all of which are tumor-bearing. Then this second interpretation of the null hypothesis specifies that the proportions of the three tumor types arising in each strain are identical.

The procedure for determining the significance level of the data in an $a \times b$ contingency table with respect to the null hypothesis, H_0, is a simple generalization of the χ^2 test for a 2×2 table. The steps in the procedure are the following:

(1) Compute a corresponding $a \times b$ table of expected numbers based on the row totals $R_1, R_2, \ldots, R_a$ and the column totals $C_1, C_2, \ldots, C_b$ in the observed table. The formula for the expected number, e_{ij}, in the cell specifying the joint category A_i and B_j is

$$e_{ij} = R_i \times \left(\frac{C_j}{N}\right) = R_i \times C_j/N.$$

Table 4.7. The $a \times b$ table of expected values corresponding to the observed data summarized in Table 4.5

Classification scheme A	Classification scheme B					Total
	B_1	B_2	$\cdot$	$\cdot$	$\cdot$	B_b	
A_1	e_{11}	e_{12}	$\cdot$	$\cdot$	$\cdot$	e_{1b}	R_1
A_2	e_{21}	e_{22}	$\cdot$	$\cdot$	$\cdot$	e_{2b}	R_2
$\cdot$	$\cdot$	$\cdot$				$\cdot$	$\cdot$
$\cdot$	$\cdot$	$\cdot$				$\cdot$	$\cdot$
$\cdot$	$\cdot$	$\cdot$				$\cdot$	$\cdot$
A_a	e_{a1}	e_{a2}	$\cdot$	$\cdot$	$\cdot$	e_{ab}	R_a
Total	C_1	C_2	$\cdot$	$\cdot$	$\cdot$	C_b	N

Notice that this number is obtained by first multiplying the unique row and column totals corresponding to the joint category A_i and B_j. The resulting product is divided by N, the overall sample size. As we indicated above, this formula for calculating e_{ij} is a simple extension of the rule which we discussed for 2×2 tables in §4.2. Recall, also, that in the 2×2 case the table of expected values could be completed by subtraction from row and column totals after calculating e_{11}. Likewise, in the $a \times b$ case, the last entry in each row and column of the table of expected numbers could be obtained by subtracting the other calculated values in the row and column from the corresponding row or column total. This means that a total of $(a-1) \times (b-1)$ values of e_{ij} could be calculated using the formula given above, and the remaining $(a+b-1)$ values can then be determined by subtraction. Table 4.7 shows the table of expected values corresponding to the $a \times b$ contingency table displayed in Table 4.5. Detailed calculations for the PAS, streptomycin clinical trial example, showing the 3×3 table of expected numbers, are given in Table 4.8.

(2) If a certain row or column in the table of expected numbers contains entries which are generally smaller than 5, it is usually wise to combine this row or column with another suitable row or column category to ensure that all of the e_{ij}'s are at least 5. Small expected numbers can seriously affect the accuracy of the approximation which is used to calculate the significance level of the data with respect to the null hypothesis. Of course, the combined

Table 4.8. The 3×3 table of expected values corresponding to the sputum analysis data summarized in Table 4.6

Treatment	Sputum analysis			Total
	positive smear	negative smear, positive culture	negative smear, negative culture	
PAS only	$\dfrac{99 \times 139}{273} = 50.41$	$\dfrac{99 \times 66}{273} = 23.93$	$\dfrac{99 \times 68}{273} = 24.66$	99
Streptomycin only	$\dfrac{84 \times 139}{273} = 42.77$	$\dfrac{84 \times 66}{273} = 20.31$	$\dfrac{84 \times 68}{273} = 20.92$	84
Combined drugs	$\dfrac{90 \times 139}{273} = 45.82$	$\dfrac{90 \times 66}{273} = 21.76$	$\dfrac{90 \times 68}{273} = 22.42$	90
Total	139	66	68	273

categories must represent a reasonable method of classification in the context of the problem.

(3) Using the two $a \times b$ tables of observed and expected numbers, calculate for each of the $a \times b$ joint categories the quantity

$$\frac{(O_{ij}-e_{ij})^2}{e_{ij}}.$$

Figure 4.1 shows a 3×3 table displaying these values for the PAS, streptomycin clinical trial.

(4) The test statistic, T, is the sum of the individual values of $(O_{ij}-e_{ij})^2/e_{ij}$ for all $a \times b$ joint categories. If we call the resulting sum t_0, then t_0 is the observed value of the test statistic. A mathematical expression which describes all this calculation is the simple formula

$$T = \sum_{i=1}^{a} \sum_{j=1}^{b} \frac{(O_{ij}-e_{ij})^2}{e_{ij}}.$$

As we explained in §4.2, the symbol $\sum_{i=1}^{a} \sum_{j=1}^{b}$ means that the $a \times b$ individual values of $(O_{ij}-e_{ij})^2/e_{ij}$ must be added together. Notice that this test statistic is similar to the one specified in §4.2 for the 2×2 table. However, the formula has been generalized to accommodate a rows and b columns. Notice,

Treatment	Sputum analysis		
	positive smear	negative smear, positive culture	negative smear, negative culture
PAS only	$\dfrac{(56-50.41)^2}{50.41} = 0.62$	$\dfrac{(30-23.93)^2}{23.93} = 1.54$	$\dfrac{(13-24.66)^2}{24.66} = 5.51$
Streptomycin only	$\dfrac{(46-42.77)^2}{42.77} = 0.24$	$\dfrac{(18-20.31)^2}{20.31} = 0.26$	$\dfrac{(20-20.92)^2}{20.92} = 0.04$
Combined drugs	$\dfrac{(37-45.82)^2}{45.82} = 1.70$	$\dfrac{(18-21.76)^2}{21.76} = 0.65$	$\dfrac{(35-22.42)^2}{22.42} = 7.06$

$t_0 = 0.62 + 1.54 + 5.51 + 0.24 + 0.26 + 0.04 + 1.70 + 0.65 + 7.06 = 17.62.$

Fig. 4.1. Calculating the quantities $(O_{ij} - e_{ij})^2/e_{ij}$ and t_0, the observed value of the test statistic, for the sputum analysis data.

also, that with the more general $a \times b$ table a continuity correction is not used.

(5) As in the case of the 2×2 table, if t_0 is the value of the test statistic for the observed data, then values of T which equal or exceed t_0, i.e., $T \geqslant t_0$, correspond to $a \times b$ contingency tables which are no more consistent with the null hypothesis, H_0, than the observed data. Therefore, the significance level of the data with respect to H_0 is obtained by calculating $\Pr(T \geqslant t_0)$. Statisticians have determined that if H_0 is true, i.e., if the A and B classification schemes are independent, then the probability distribution of T is approximately the same as that of a χ_k^2 (chi-squared with k degrees of freedom) random variable. The value of k depends on the number of rows and columns in the rectangular contingency table; more specifically, $k = (a-1) \times (b-1)$, the number of expected values which were necessarily obtained by the multiplication rule $e_{ij} = R_i \times C_j/N$. By referring to the statistical tables for the χ^2 family of distributions, we can calculate the probability that $\chi_k^2 \geqslant t_0$; for details regarding this calculation, see §4.4. Therefore, the significance level of the data with respect to the null hypothesis is approximately $\Pr(\chi_k^2 \geqslant t_0)$, where t_0 represents the value of the test statistic, T, for the observed data.

Figure 4.1 not only displays the nine individual values of the quantity $(O_{ij}-e_{ij})^2/e_{ij}$ but also gives the observed value of T, namely $t_0 = 17.62$. Since the contingency table from which t_o was derived consisted of three rows ($a=3$) and three columns ($b=3$), the distribution of T, if H_0 is true, is χ_4^2. Therefore, the significance level of the data is given by $Pr(\chi_4^2 \geqslant 17.62)$. Statistical tables for the χ^2 distribution show that this probability is less than 0.005. Therefore, we conclude that the data contradict the null hypothesis of independence, i.e., patient condition at the conclusion of the clinical trial seemingly is associated with the type of treatment received.

Notice that the expected numbers in the 3×3 table presented in Table 4.8 were all larger than 5. In this case it was not necessary to combine rows or columns in order to improve the accuracy of the approximate significance test. However, the following example will illustrate more precisely what is involved when too many of the expected numbers are too small.

In a prospective study of venocclusive disease (VOD) of the liver, *McDonald* et al. [1984] reviewed the records of 255 patients undergoing bone marrow transplant for malignancy. A primary purpose of the study was to investigate the relationship between pretransplant liver disease and the incidence of VOD. The patients were divided into five diagnosis groups: D_1 (primarily acute lymphocytic leukemia), D_2 (primarily acute myelogenous leukemia), D_3 (chronic myelogenous leukemia), D_4 (solid tumors) and D_5 (lymphoma, lymphosarcoma and Hodgkin's disease). Preliminary analysis of the data revealed that both pretransplant SGOT (aspartate aminotransferase) and diagnosis group were associated with the incidence of VOD. In order to determine whether SGOT level and diagnosis were associated with respect to VOD, the cross-tabulation presented in Table 4.9a was prepared. If SGOT levels and diagnosis group are independent, the expected values which are given in parentheses involve too many small values to carry out a reliable test of the null hypothesis of independence. However, combining the diagnosis groups D_4 and D_5, and also the SGOT categories 2–3$\times$, 3–4$\times$ and >4$\times$ Normal results in a 3×4 table with larger expected numbers in many of the cells (see Table 4.9b). Notice, too, that in general, the observed and expected numbers agree fairly closely in the cells which disappear through the combining of rows and columns. The observed value of the test statistic, T, was calculated for the revised table and its value was determined to be $t_o = 4.52$. Since the revised table has three rows ($a=3$) and four columns ($b=4$), the approximate χ^2 distribution of T has $2 \times 3 = 6$ degrees of freedom. Therefore, the significance level of the data with respect to the null hypothesis of independence is $Pr(\chi_6^2 \geqslant 4.52)$, which exceeds 0.25. Therefore, the final conclusion of this analysis is that, with respect to VOD, pretransplant SGOT levels and patient diagnosis are not related.

Table 4.9. SGOT levels and diagnosis data for 255 patients transplanted for malignancy: (a) initial tabulation; (b) revised tabulation

a Initial tabulation

SGOT levels	Diagnosis group					Total
	D_1	D_2	D_3	D_4	D_5	
Normal	70 (64.45)[1]	70 (72.91)	14 (15.62)	9 (9.11)	3 (3.91)	166
1–2 × Normal	14 (18.25)	21 (20.64)	7 (4.42)	3 (2.58)	2 (1.11)	47
2–3 × Normal	3 (5.44)	8 (6.15)	2 (1.32)	1 (0.77)	0 (0.32)	14
3–4 × Normal	3 (3.88)	6 (4.39)	1 (0.94)	0 (0.55)	0 (0.24)	10
> 4 × Normal	9 (6.98)	7 (7.91)	0 (1.70)	1 (0.99)	1 (0.42)	18
Total	99	112	24	14	6	255

b Revised tabulation

SGOT levels	Diagnosis group				Total
	D_1	D_2	D_3	D_4 and D_5	
Normal	70 (64.45)[1]	70 (72.91)	14 (15.62)	12 (13.02)	166
1–2 × Normal	14 (18.25)	21 (20.64)	7 (4.42)	5 (3.69)	47
> 2 × Normal	15 (16.30)	21 (18.45)	3 (3.96)	3 (3.29)	42
Total	99	112	24	20	255

[1] The values in parentheses are expected numbers if the row and column classifications are independent.

4.4. Using Statistical Tables of the χ^2 Probability Distribution

In §1.2 we introduced the idea that, if X is a continuous random variable, probabilities for X are represented by the area under the corresponding probability curve and above an interval of values for X. The χ^2 family of probability distributions is a set of continuous random variables with similar, but distinct, probability curves. Each member of the family is uniquely identified by the value of a positive parameter, k, which is known, historically, as the 'degrees of freedom' of the distribution. This indexing parameter, k, is usually attached to the χ^2 symbol as a subscript. For example, χ_4^2 identifies the χ^2 probability distribution which has four degrees of freedom. A sketch of the χ_4^2, χ_7^2 and χ_{10}^2 probability curves is given in Figure 4.2a. Although the indexing parameter k is always called degrees of freedom, it can be shown that the mean of χ_k^2 is exactly k and the variance is 2k. Therefore, we could choose to identify χ_4^2, for example, as the χ^2 probability distribution with mean four. However, convention dictates that it should be called the χ^2 distribution with four degrees of freedom.

Thus far, the only reason we have required the χ^2 probability distribution has been the calculation of significance levels for the approximate test in 2×2 or larger contingency tables. In §4.2 we learned that if t_o is the observed value of the test statistic T, then the significance level of the corresponding null hypothesis is approximately $\Pr(\chi_1^2 \geq t_o)$. Similarly, in §4.3 we discovered that if t_o is the observed value of the test statistic computed for an $a \times b$ contingency table, then the significance level of the corresponding null hypothesis is approximately $\Pr(\chi_k^2 \geq t_o)$, where $k = (a-1) \times (b-1)$. Judging from these uses for the χ^2 distribution, we require tables for each possible χ^2 probability distribution, i.e., each value of k, the degrees of freedom. These tables should specify the area under the χ_k^2 probability curve which corresponds to the interval $\chi_k^2 \geq t_o$; such intervals are known as right-hand tail probabilities. And since we cannot predict values of t_o in advance, we seemingly require a table for every possible value of t_o. Since this would require a separate statistical table for every degree of freedom, it would appear that χ^2 tables must be very unwieldy.

Although sets of χ^2 tables do exist which follow the pattern we have described above, a much more compact version has been devised, and these are usually quite adequate. Since the significance level of the χ^2 test is approximate, it is frequently satisfactory to know a narrow range within which the approximate significance level of a test lies. It follows that, for any member of the χ^2 family of probability distributions, we only require a dozen or so special reference points, called critical values. These are values of the random variable which correspond to specified significance levels or, equivalently, values which cut off predetermined amounts of probability (area) in the right-hand tail of the probability curve. For example, we might wish to know the critical values for χ_4^2 which correspond to the right-hand tail probabilities 0.5, 0.25, 0.10, 0.05, 0.025, 0.01 and 0.005. The actual numbers which correspond to these probability levels for χ_4^2 are 3.357, 5.385, 7.779, 9.488, 11.14, 13.28 and 14.86. Figure 4.2b shows a sketch of the χ_4^2 probability curve indicating the location of these critical values and the corresponding right-

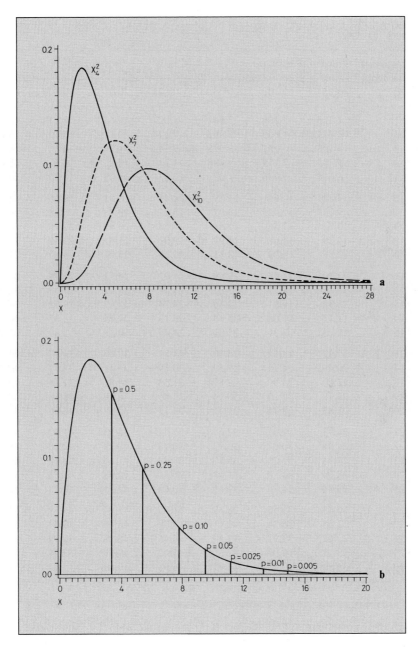

Fig. 4.2. Chi-squared probability curves. **a** χ_4^2, χ_7^2 and χ_{10}^2. **b** The location of selected critical values for χ_4^2.

Table 4.10. Critical values of the χ^2 distribution; the table gives values of the number t_o such that $Pr(\chi_k^2 \geq t_o) = p$

Degrees of freedom (k)	Probability level, p						
	0.25	0.10	0.05	0.025	0.01	0.005	0.001
1	1.323	2.706	3.841	5.024	6.635	7.879	10.83
2	2.773	4.605	5.991	7.378	9.210	10.60	13.82
3	4.108	6.251	7.815	9.348	11.34	12.84	16.27
4	5.385	7.779	9.488	11.14	13.28	14.86	18.47
5	6.626	9.236	11.07	12.83	15.09	16.75	20.52
6	7.841	10.64	12.59	14.45	16.81	18.55	22.46
7	9.037	12.02	14.07	16.01	18.48	20.28	24.32
8	10.22	13.36	15.51	17.53	20.09	21.96	26.13
9	11.39	14.68	16.92	19.02	21.67	23.59	27.88
10	12.55	15.99	18.31	20.48	23.21	25.19	29.59
11	13.70	17.28	19.68	21.92	24.72	26.76	31.26
12	14.85	18.55	21.03	23.34	26.22	28.30	32.91
13	15.98	19.81	22.36	24.74	27.69	29.82	34.53
14	17.12	21.06	23.68	26.12	29.14	31.32	36.12
15	18.25	22.31	25.00	27.49	30.58	32.80	37.70
16	19.37	23.54	26.30	28.85	32.00	34.27	39.25
17	20.49	24.77	27.59	30.19	33.41	35.72	40.79
18	21.60	25.99	28.87	31.53	34.81	37.16	42.31
19	22.72	27.20	30.14	32.85	36.19	38.58	43.82
20	23.83	28.41	31.41	34.17	37.57	40.00	45.32
21	24.93	29.62	32.67	35.48	38.93	41.40	46.80
22	26.04	30.81	33.92	36.78	40.29	42.80	48.27
23	27.14	32.01	35.17	38.08	41.64	44.18	49.73
24	28.24	33.20	36.42	39.36	42.98	45.56	51.18
25	29.34	34.38	37.65	40.65	44.31	46.93	52.62
26	30.43	35.56	38.89	41.92	45.64	48.29	54.05
27	31.53	36.74	40.11	43.19	46.96	49.64	55.48
28	32.62	37.92	41.34	44.46	48.28	50.99	56.89
29	33.71	39.09	42.56	45.72	49.59	52.34	58.30
30	34.80	40.26	43.77	46.98	50.89	53.67	59.70

hand tail probabilities. Such a table requires only one line of critical values for each degree of freedom. Thus, an entire set of tables for the χ^2 family of probability distributions can be presented on a single page. This is the method of presentation which most χ^2 tables adopt, and an example of χ^2 statistical tables which follow this format is reproduced in Table 4.10. The rows of the table correspond to different values of k, the degrees of freedom parameter. The columns identify predetermined right-hand tail probabilities, i.e., 0.25, 0.05, 0.01, etc., and the entries in the table specify the corresponding critical values for the χ^2 probability distribution identified by its unique degrees of freedom.

The actual use of χ^2 tables is very straightforward. In order to calculate $\Pr(\chi_k^2 \geqslant t_o)$, locate the row for k degrees of freedom. In that row, find the two numbers, say t_L and t_U, which are closest to t_o so that $t_L \leqslant t_o \leqslant t_U$. For example, if we want to evaluate $\Pr(\chi_4^2 \geqslant 10.4)$ these numbers are $t_L = 9.488$ and $t_U = 11.14$ since $9.488 < 10.4 < 11.14$. Since $t_L = 9.488$ corresponds to a right-hand tail probability of 0.05 and $t_U = 11.14$ corresponds to a right-hand tail probability of 0.025, it follows that $\Pr(\chi_4^2 \geqslant 10.4)$ is smaller than 0.05 and larger than 0.025, i.e., $0.05 > \Pr(\chi_4^2 \geqslant 10.4) > 0.025$. And if $\Pr(\chi_4^2 \geqslant 10.4)$ is the approximate significance level of a test, then we know that the p-value of the test is between 0.025 and 0.05.

5 Some Warnings concerning 2 × 2 Tables

5.1. Introduction

In the two preceding chapters, we discussed a significance test for 2×2 tables such as the one shown in Table 5.1. Although this version of a 2×2 table contains different symbols for the row totals, column totals and cell entries, the change in notation considerably simplifies the presentation of the two topics addressed in this chapter.

As the title suggests, the use of either Fisher's test or the χ^2 test to analyze a set of data is so straightforward that researchers are tempted to use one test or the other even when the use of either test is not appropriate. As a cautionary note then, in this chapter we intend to identify two situations which appear tailor-made for 2×2 tables but which, in fact, properly require a modified analysis. The first situation concerns the issue of combining 2×2 tables, while the second problem involves the proper method for analyzing paired binary data. In each case, the principles which are involved, namely stratification and pairing, are important statistical concepts which also apply to many other methods for analyzing data.

5.2. Combining 2 × 2 Tables

Both Fisher's test (chapter 3) and the χ^2 test outlined in chapter 4 determine the degree to which the data summarized in a 2×2 table are consistent with the null hypothesis that the probability of success is the same in two distinct groups. The two important assumptions of either test which we noted previously are that the probability of success must be the same for each subject in a group, and that the outcome of the experiment for any subject may not influence the outcome for any member of either group.

Unfortunately, the first of these assumptions, namely that the probability of success is the same for each member of a group, is often not true; there

Table 5.1. A 2 × 2 table summarizing binary data collected from two groups

	Success	Failure	Total
Group 1	a	A – a	A
Group 2	b	B – b	B
Total	r	N – r	N

may be factors other than group membership which influence the probability of success. If the effect of such factors is ignored and the observed data are summarized in a single 2 × 2 table, the test of significance that is used to analyze the data could mask important effects or generate spurious ones, as the following example illustrates.

A study of the effect of prenatal care on fetal mortality was undertaken in two different clinics; the results of the study are summarized, by clinic, in Figure 5.1a. Clearly, there is no evidence in the data from either clinic to suggest that the probability or rate of fetal mortality varies with the amount of prenatal care delivered. However, if we ignore the fact that this rate is roughly three times higher in Clinic 2 and combine the data in the single 2 × 2 table shown in Figure 5.1b, the combined data support the opposite conclusion. Why? Notice that in Clinic 1 there are fewer deaths overall and much more intensive care, while in Clinic 2 there are more deaths and much less intensive care. Therefore, the significant difference in the two rates of fetal mortality observed in the combined table is due to the very large number of more intensive care patients contributed by Clinic 1 with its low death rate.

The preceding example illustrates only one of the possible hazards of combining 2 × 2 tables. If there are other factors, in addition to the characteristic of major interest, which might affect the probability of success, then it is important to adjust for these other factors, which are sometimes called confounding factors, in analyzing the data. In the preceding example, the primary focus of the study is the relationship between the amount of prenatal care and the rate of fetal mortality. However, we observed that the amount of prenatal care received depended on the additional factor representing clinic location (Clinic 1 or Clinic 2) which also influenced the rate of fetal mortality. Thus, clinic location is a confounding factor. To properly assess the relation-

a

Prenatal care	Clinic 1		Clinic 2	
	L	M	L	M
Died	12	16	34	4
Survived	176	293	197	23
Total	188	309	231	27
Fetal mortality rate	0.064	0.055	0.173	0.174
Observed value of T for χ^2 test	$t_o = 0.13$		$t_o = 0.09$	
Significance level of χ^2 test	> 0.50		> 0.75	

b

Prenatal care	L	M
Died	46	20
Survived	373	316
Total	419	336
Fetal mortality rate	0.11	0.06
Observed value of T for χ^2 test	$t_o = 5.29$	
Significance level of χ^2 test	< 0.025	

Fig. 5.1. Details of the analysis of a study of fetal mortality and the amount of prenatal health care delivered (L ≡ less, M ≡ more). **a** By individual clinic. **b** Combining over clinics.

ship between amount of prenatal care and fetal mortality, it was necessary to separately consider the data for each clinic. This simple technique of separately investigating the primary question for different cases of a confounding factor is known as stratifying the data; thus, to adjust the analysis of the study for the possible confusion which clinic location would have introduced, the study data were stratified by clinic location, i.e., divided into the data from Clinic 1 and the data from Clinic 2. Whenever it is thought necessary to adjust the analysis of a 2 × 2 table for possible confounding factors, the simplest way to effect this adjustment is to stratify the study data according to the

Table 5.2. A 2 × 2 table summarizing the binary data for level i of a confounding factor

	Confounding factor level i		Total
	success	failure	
Group 1	a_i	$A_i - a_i$	A_i
Group 2	b_i	$B_i - b_i$	B_i
Total	r_i	$N_i - r_i$	N_i

different cases of the possible confounding factor or factors. Suppose, for the sake of illustration, that there are a total of k distinct cases (statisticians often call these cases 'levels') for a possible confounding factor, e.g., k different clinics participating in the fetal mortality and prenatal care study. Stratifying the study data on the basis of this confounding factor will give us k distinct 2 × 2 tables like the one shown in Table 5.2, where the possible values of i, representing the distinct levels of the confounding factor, would be the numbers 1 through k.

As we saw in chapter 4, the χ^2 test for a single 2 × 2 table evaluates the discrepancy between the observed and expected values for each cell in the table, assuming that the row and column totals are fixed and the probability of success in the two groups is the same. The test of significance which correctly combines the results in all k stratified 2 × 2 tables calculates, for each distinct 2 × 2 table, an expected value, e_i, corresponding to a_i; this expected value, e_i, is based on the usual assumptions that the row and column totals A_i, B_i, r_i and $N_i - r_i$ are fixed and that the probability of success in the two groups is the same. Notice, however, that the probability of success may now vary from one stratum (2 × 2 table) to another; the test no longer requires that the probability of success must be the same for each level of the confounding factor. Instead, the null hypothesis for this test of significance specifies that, for each distinct level of the confounding factor, the probabilities of success for Groups 1 and 2 must be the same; however, this hypothesis does allow the common probabilities of success to differ from one level of the confounding factor to another. In terms of the fetal mortality example, the null hypothesis requires a constant fetal mortality rate in Clinic 1, regardless of prenatal care received, and a constant, but possibly different, fetal mortality rate in Clinic 2, regardless of prenatal care received.

2×2 Table

Prenatal care	Clinic 1			Clinic 2		
	L	M	Total	L	M	Total
Died	$12 = a_1$	16	$28 = A_1$	$34 = a_2$	4	$38 = A_2$
Survived	176	293	$469 = B_1$	197	23	$220 = B_2$
Total	$188 = r_1$	309	$497 = N_1$	$231 = r_2$	27	$258 = N_2$

Observed value	$a_1 = 12$		$a_2 = 34$
Expected value	$e_1 = \dfrac{188 \times 28}{497} = 10.59$		$e_2 = \dfrac{231 \times 38}{258} = 34.02$
Variance	$V_1 = \dfrac{188 \times 309 \times 28 \times 469}{497^2 \times 496} = 6.23$		$V_2 = \dfrac{231 \times 27 \times 38 \times 220}{258^2 \times 257} = 3.05$

$O = 12 + 34 = 46, \quad E = 10.59 + 34.02 = 44.61, \quad V = 6.23 + 3.05 = 9.28$

$$t_0 = \frac{(|46 - 44.61| - \frac{1}{2})^2}{9.28} = 0.09$$

Fig. 5.2. Details of the correct analysis of the fetal mortality data, adjusting for the confounding effect of clinic location.

Of course, evaluating the expected numbers $e_1, e_2, \ldots, e_k$ automatically determines the corresponding expected values for the remaining three cells in each of the k distinct 2×2 tables. As we might anticipate, the test statistic evaluates the discrepancy between the sum of the k observed values, $O = a_1 + a_2 + \ldots + a_k = \sum_{i=1}^{k} a_i$, and the sum of the corresponding k expected values, $E = e_1 + e_2 + \ldots + e_k = \sum_{i=1}^{k} e_i$. To determine the significance level of the test we need to compute:

(1) $O = \sum_{i=1}^{k} a_i, \quad E = \sum_{i=1}^{k} e_i$ where $e_i = r_i A_i / N_i$;

(2) $V = V_1 + V_2 + \ldots + V_k = \sum_{i=1}^{k} V_i$ where $V_i = \dfrac{r_i (N_i - r_i) A_i B_i}{N_i^2 (N_i - 1)}$;

(3) the observed value, say t_0, of the test statistic

$$T = \frac{(|O - E| - \frac{1}{2})^2}{V}.$$

The details of these calculations for the fetal mortality study we have been discussing are given in Figure 5.2. For this set of data the observed value of the test statistic, T, is $t_o = 0.09$.

If the null hypothesis is true, the test statistic, T, has a distribution which is approximately χ_1^2. Therefore, the significance level of the test, which is $Pr(T \geqslant t_o)$, can be determined by evaluating the probability that $\chi_1^2 \geqslant t_o$, i.e., $Pr(\chi_1^2 \geqslant t_o)$. In the case of the fetal mortality study, the approximate significance level is $Pr(\chi_1^2 \geqslant 0.09) > 0.25$. Therefore, after adjusting the analysis for the confounding effect of clinic location, we conclude that there is no evidence in the data to suggest that the rate of fetal mortality is associated with the amount of prenatal care received.

Much more has been written about the hazards of combining 2 × 2 tables. For example, an exact test of the null hypothesis we have just discussed can be performed. However, the details of that version of the test are beyond the intent and scope of this brief discussion. In our view, it suffices to alert the reader to the hazards involved. For situations more complicated than the one which we have outlined, we suggest consulting a statistician.

5.3. Matched Pairs Binary Data

A second situation which, at first glance, seems tailored to the straightforward use of Fisher's test or the χ^2 test of significance in a 2 × 2 table is that of binary data which incorporate matching. The following example illustrates more precisely the situation we have in mind.

Two pathologists each examine coded material from the same 100 tumors and classify the material as malignant or benign. The investigator conducting the study is interested in determining the extent to which the pathologists differ in their assessments of the study material. The results could be recorded in the 2 × 2 table shown in Table 5.3a.

Although the data are presented in the form of a 2 × 2 table, certain facets of the study have been obscured. The total number of tumors involved appears to be 200, but in fact there were only 100. Also, some tumors will be more clearly malignant than the rest; therefore, the assumption that there is a constant probability of malignancy being coded for each tumor is unreasonable. Finally, the table omits important information about the tumors which A and B classified in the same way and those on which they differed.

A better presentation of the study results might be the 2 × 2 table shown in Table 5.3b, but this is still not a 2 × 2 table to which we could properly

Table 5.3. The results of a study to determine the extent of agreement between two pathologists: **(a)** initial tabulation; **(b)** revised presentation

a Initial tabulation

	Malignant	Benign	Total
Pathologist A	18	82	100
Pathologist B	10	90	100
Total	28	172	200

b Revised presentation

Pathologist B	Pathologist A		Total
	malignant	benign	
Malignant	9	1	10
Benign	9	81	90
Total	18	82	100

apply either Fisher's test or the χ^2 test of significance discussed in chapters 3 and 4. Though the observations are independent (there are exactly 100 tumors, each classified by A and by B), it is still unreasonable to suppose that for each of B's malignant tumors, and separately for each of B's benign tumors, there is a constant probability that A will identify the same material as malignant. Nevertheless, this is one of the two principal assumptions of both the χ^2 test and Fisher's test. (Recall that, within each group, the probability of success must be constant. In this example, the two groups are B's malignant and benign tumors.)

An appropriate way to present and analyze these data is as a series of 2 × 2 tables, with each table recording the experimental results for one tumor. A sample 2 × 2 table is shown in Table 5.4. It should be immediately apparent that the method for analyzing this series of 2 × 2 tables is the procedure described in the preceding section. Because the study material is so variable, each sample item represents a distinct case of the confounding factor 'tumor material'. Therefore, we need to analyze the study by adjusting the

Table 5.4. A 2×2 table indicating the conclusion of each pathologist concerning tumor sample i

	Malignant	Benign	Total
Pathologist A	a_i	$A_i - a_i$	$A_i = 1$
Pathologist B	b_i	$B_i - b_i$	$B_i = 1$
Total	r_i	$N_i - r_i$	$N_i = 2$

analysis for the confounding effect of tumor material. If we do this, the 90 2×2 tables which correspond to tumors on which the pathologists were agreed contribute nothing to the numerator, $(|O-E|-\frac{1}{2})^2$, and denominator, V, of the test statistic

$$T = \frac{(|O-E|-\frac{1}{2})^2}{V}.$$

This occurs because whenever the pathologists agree, either $a_i = 1$, $e_i = 1$, $r_i = 2$ and $N_i - r_i = 2-2 = 0$ or $a_i = 0$, $e_i = 0$, $r_i = 0$ and $N_i - r_i = 2-0 = 2$, i.e., the net contribution to O−E is either $1-1 = 0$ or $0-0 = 0$ and $V_i = 0$ in both cases since one of r_i, $N_i - r_i$ is always zero. Thus, only information from 'discordant pairs' contributes to a test of the null hypothesis that the two pathologists do not differ in their assessment of tumors. A moment's reflection will verify that if the pathologists were in total agreement, there would be no statistical evidence to contradict the null hypothesis; therefore, it makes sense that only disagreements should provide possible evidence to the contrary.

As a final, cautionary note we add that care should be exercised in using the test statistic, T, with matched pairs binary data. A rough rule-of-thumb specifies that there should be at least ten disagreements or discordant pairs. For situations involving fewer than ten, there is a fairly simple calculation which yields the exact significance level of the test, and we suggest consulting a statistician in these circumstances. For the example we have been discussing, the exact significance level of a test of the null hypothesis that there is no disagreement between the pathologists is 0.0215. On the other hand, if we use the test statistic, T, it turns out that $O = 9$, $E = 5$ and $V = 2.5$; therefore, the observed value of T is

$$t_0 = \frac{(|9-5|-\frac{1}{2})^2}{2.5} = 4.90.$$

According to Table 4.10, the 0.05 and 0.025 critical values for the χ_1^2 probability distribution are 3.84 and 5.02, respectively. Therefore, we know that the approximate significance level of the test is between 0.025 and 0.05. This compares favorably with the exact value of 0.0215 which we quoted previously.

Though we have not, by any means, exhausted the subject of analyzing binary data, at the same time not all data are binary in nature. While interested readers may wish to divert their attention to more advanced treatments of this subject, we continue our exposition of statistical methods used in medical research by discussing, in chapter 6, the presentation and analysis of survival data.

6 Kaplan-Meier or 'Actuarial' Survival Curves

6.1. Introduction

In medical research, it is often useful to display a summary of the survival experience of a group of patients. We can do this conceptually by considering the specified group of patients as a random sample from a much larger population of similar patients. Then the survival experience of the available patients describes, in general terms, what we might expect for any patient in the larger population.

In chapter 1, we briefly introduced the cumulative probability function. With survival data, it is convenient to use a related function called the survival function, $\Pr(T > t)$. If T is a random variable representing survival time, then the survival function, $\Pr(T > t)$, is the probability that T exceeds t units. Since the cumulative probability function is $\Pr(T \leqslant t)$, these two functions are related via the equation

$$\Pr(T > t) = 1 - \Pr(T \leqslant t).$$

If $\Pr(T > t)$ is the survival function for a specified population of patients, then, by using a random sample of survival times from that population, we would like to *estimate* the survival function. The concept of estimation, based on a random sample, is central to statistics, and other examples of estimation will be discussed in later chapters. Here we proceed with a very specific discussion of the estimation of survival functions.

A graphical presentation of a survival function is frequently the most convenient. In this form it is sometimes referred to as a survival curve. Figure 6.1 presents the estimated survival curve for 31 individuals diagnosed with lymphoma and presenting with clinical symptoms. The horizontal axis represents time since diagnosis and the vertical axis represents the probability or chance of survival, expressed as a percentage. For example, based on this group of 31 patients, we would estimate that 60% of similar patients should survive at least one year, but less than 40% should survive for three years or more following diagnosis.

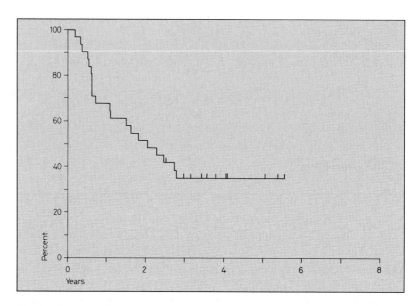

Fig. 6.1. The estimated survival curve for 31 patients diagnosed with lymphoma and presenting with clinical symptoms.

The estimation of survival curves like the one presented in Figure 6.1 is one of the oldest methods of analyzing survival data. The early methodology is due to *Berkson and Gage* [1950], and is also discussed by *Cutler and Ederer* [1958]. Their method is appropriate when survival times are grouped into intervals and the number of individuals dying in each interval is recorded. This approach also allows for the possibility that individuals may be lost to follow-up in an interval. Such events give rise to censored survival times, which are different from observed survival times. Survival curves based on the methodology of *Berkson and Gage* are frequently referred to as 'actuarial' curves because the techniques used parallel those employed by actuaries.

The grouping of survival times may be useful for illustrative and computational purposes. However, with the increased access to computers which has emerged in recent years, it is now common practice to base an analysis on precise survival times rather than grouped data.

Figure 6.1 actually displays a 'Kaplan-Meier' (K-M) estimate of a survival curve. This estimate was first proposed in 1958 by *Kaplan and Meier*. The K-M estimate is also frequently called an actuarial estimate, because it is closely related to the earlier methods. In this chapter, we will restrict ourselves to a discussion of the Kaplan-Meier estimate in order to illustrate the most important concepts. We will consistently use survival time as the variable of interest, although the methodology can be used to describe time to any well-defined endpoint, for example, relapse.

6.2. General Features of the Kaplan-Meier Estimate

If we have recorded the survival times for n individuals and r of these times exceed a specified time t, then a natural estimate of the probability of surviving more than t units would be r/n. This is the estimate which would be derived from a Kaplan-Meier estimated survival curve. However, the Kaplan-Meier methodology extends this natural estimate to the situation when not all the survival times are known exactly. If an individual has only been observed for t units and death has not occurred, then we say that this individual has a censored survival time; all we know is that the individual's survival time must exceed t units. In order to illustrate the general features of the Kaplan-Meier estimate, including the methodology appropriate for censored survival times, we consider the following simple example.

Figure 6.2a presents data from a hypothetical study in which ten patients were enrolled. The observations represent the time, in days, from treatment to death. Five patients were observed to die and the remaining five have censored survival times. From these data we intend to construct an estimate of the survival curve for the study population.

Although one observation is censored at Day 1, no patients are recorded as dying prior to Day 3 following treatment. Therefore, we estimate that no deaths are likely to occur prior to Day 3 and say that the probability of surviving for at least three days is 1. As before, we use the symbol $Pr(T > t)$ to represent the probability that T, the survival time from treatment to death, exceeds t units. Based on the study data, we would estimate that $Pr(T > t) = 1$ for all values of t less than three days.

Nine individuals have been observed for at least three days, with one death recorded at Day 3. Therefore, the natural estimate of $Pr(T > 3)$, the probability of surviving more than three days, is 8/9. Since no deaths were recorded between Days 3 and 5, this estimate of 8/9 will apply to $Pr(T > t)$ for all values of t between Day 3 and Day 5 as well.

At Day 5 following treatment, two deaths are recorded among the seven patients who have been observed for at least five days. Therefore, among patients who survive until Day 5, the natural estimate of the probability of surviving for more than five days is 5/7. However, this is not an estimate of

Pr(T > 5) for all patients, but only for those who have already survived until Day 5. The probability of survival beyond Day 5 is equal to the probability of survival until Day 5 multiplied by the probability of survival beyond Day 5 for patients who survive until Day 5. Based on the natural estimates from our hypothetical study, this product is $\frac{8}{9} \times \frac{5}{7} = \frac{40}{63}$. This multiplication of probabilities characterizes the calculation of a Kaplan-Meier estimated survival curve.

No further deaths are recorded in our example until Day 7, so that the estimate 40/63 corresponds to Pr(T > t) for all values of t between Day 5 and Day 7.

Four individuals in the study were followed until Day 7; two of these died at Day 7, one is censored at Day 7 and one is observed until Day 8. It is customary to assume that when an observed survival time and a censored survival time have the same recorded value, the censored survival time is larger than the observed survival time. Therefore, the estimate of survival beyond Day 7 for those patients alive until Day 7 would be 2/4. Since the estimate of survival until Day 7 is 40/63, the overall estimate of survival beyond Day 7 is $\frac{40}{63} \times \frac{2}{4} = \frac{20}{63}$, and so the estimate of Pr(T > t) is $\frac{20}{63}$ for all values of t exceeding 7 and during which at least one patient has been observed. The largest observation in the study is eight days; therefore Pr(T > t) = 20/63 for all values of t between Day 7 and Day 8. Since we have no information concerning survival after Day 8, we cannot estimate the survival curve beyond that point. However, if the last patient had been observed to die at Day 8, then the natural estimate of the probability of survival beyond Day 8 for individuals surviving until Day 8 would be zero (0/1). In this case, the estimated survival curve would drop to zero at Day 8 and equal zero for all values of t exceeding 8.

Figure 6.2b presents the Kaplan-Meier estimated probability of survival function for our hypothetical example. The graph of the function has horizontal sections, with vertical steps at the observed survival times; the short vertical strokes indicate the times of censored observations. This staircase appearance may not seem very realistic, since the probability of survival function for a population is generally thought to decrease smoothly with time. Nevertheless, we have not observed any deaths in the intervals between the changes in the estimated function, so that the staircase appearance is the form most consistent with our data. If we had been able to observe more survival times, the steps in our estimated function would become smaller and smaller, and the graph would more closely resemble a smooth curve.

The staircase appearance, the drop to zero if the largest observation corresponds to a death, and the undefined nature of the estimated probability

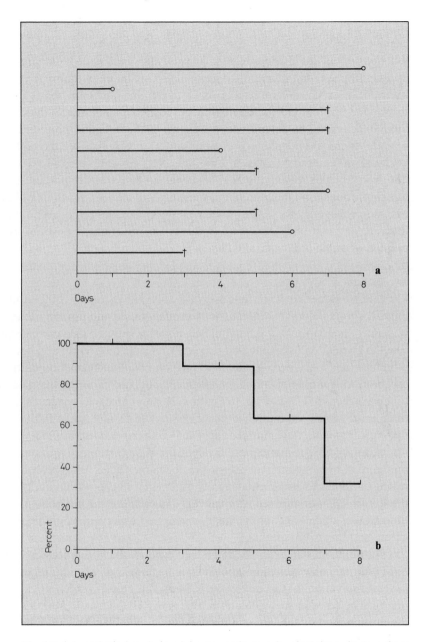

Fig. 6.2. A hypothetical study involving ten patients. **a** Survival times, in days, from treatment to death († ≡ death, ○ ≡ censored). **b** The Kaplan-Meier estimated probability of survival function.

if the largest observation time is censored, may appear to be undesirable characteristics of the Kaplan-Meier estimate of the probability of survival function. All of these features arise because the methodology attempts to estimate the survival function for a population without assuming anything regarding its expected nature, and using only a finite number of observations to provide information for estimation purposes. In some sense, therefore, these undesirable characteristics are artefacts of the statistical procedure. In practical terms, these features present no serious problems since their effects are most pronounced at points in time when very few individuals have been observed. For this reason, it would be unwise to derive any important medical conclusions from the behavior of the estimated survival function at these time points. Overall, the Kaplan-Meier estimate provides a very useful summary of survival experience and deserves its pre-eminent position as a method of displaying survival data.

Comments:

(a) One rather common summary of survival experience is the sample median survival time. This statistic is probably used more widely than is warranted; nevertheless, it is a useful benchmark. Censored data can complicate the calculation of the median survival time and, as a result, a variety of estimates can be defined. A simple indication of the median survival time can be read from a Kaplan-Meier estimated survival curve as the specific time t at which $\Pr(T > t) = 0.5$. In Figure 6.2b, this value may be identified as the time at which the estimated curve changes from more than 0.5 to less than 0.5. However, the estimated curve may be horizontal at the 0.5 level, in which case no unique number can be identified as the estimated median. The midpoint of the time interval over which the curve equals 0.5 is probably as reasonable an estimated median as any other choice in this situation. Use of the Kaplan-Meier estimated survival curve to estimate the median survival time ensures that correct use is made of censored observations in the calculation, and this is important.

As we noted earlier, if the largest observation has been censored, the K-M estimate can never equal zero and will be undefined when t exceeds this largest observation. In this case, if the K-M estimate always exceeds 0.5, then there can be no estimated median survival time. All that can be stated is that the median exceeds the largest observation.

(b) Another peculiar feature of the K-M estimated survival curve, especially at more distant times on the horizontal axis, is the presence of long horizontal lines, indicating no change in the estimated survival probability over a long period of time. It is very tempting to regard these flat portions as evidence of a 'cured fraction' of patients or a special group characterized in a similar way. Usually, these horizontal sections arise because only a few individuals were still under observation, and no particular importance should be ascribed to these 'long tails'. If the existence of such a special group of patients, such as a cured fraction, is thought to be likely, then it would be wise to consult a statistician concerning specialized methods for examining this hypothesis.

. (c) Part of the problem discussed in (b) is due to the fact that most K-M estimated survival curves are presented without any indication of the potential error in the estimate. However, a standard error for the estimated survival probability at a particular time t can be calculated, and often appears in a computer listing of the calculations relating to a Kaplan-Meier curve. A range of plausible values for the estimated probability at t units is the estimate plus or minus twice the standard error (see chapter 8). It is essential to indicate an interval such as this one if any important conclusions are to be deduced from the K-M estimate.

A very rough estimate of the standard error is given by *Peto* et al. [1977]. If the estimated survival probability at t units is p and n individuals are still under observation, then the estimated standard error is $p\sqrt{(1-p)/n}$. Since this is an approximate formula, it is possible that the range of plausible values $p \pm 2p\sqrt{(1-p)/n}$ may not lie entirely between 0 and 1; recall that all probabilities fall between these limits. If this overlap represents a serious problem, then it would be wise to consult a statistician.

(d) A critical factor in the calculation of the K-M estimated survival curve is the assumption that the reason an observation has been censored is independent of or unrelated to the cause of death. This assumption is true, for example, if censoring occurs because an individual has only been included in a trial for a specified period of observation and is still being followed. If individuals who responded poorly to a treatment were dropped from a study before death and identified as censored observations, then the K-M estimated survival curve would not be appropriate because the independent censoring assumption has been violated.

There is no good way to adjust for inappropriate censoring so it should, if possible, be avoided. Perhaps the most frequent example of this problem is censoring due to causes of death other than the particular cause which is under study. Unless the different causes of death act independently (and this assumption cannot be tested in most cases), the production of a K-M estimated survival curve corresponding to a specific cause is unwise. Methodology which is closely related to the techniques for producing K-M estimated survival curves does exist to handle this cause-specific situation, but interpretation of the estimated curves is not straightforward and statistical help is advised.

(e) Corresponding to the K-M estimated survival curve presented in Figure 6.1, Table 6.1 shows typical information provided by computer programs which calculate Kaplan-Meier estimated survival curves. Each line of the table records a survival time, the number of deaths which occurred at that time, the number of individuals under observation at that time, the K-M estimate of the probability of surviving beyond that time, and a standard error of the estimate. Typically, the standard error will not be the simple estimate of comment (c), but generally a better one involving more detailed calculations.

Table 6.1. A typical tabulation for a Kaplan-Meier survival curve; the data represent 31 lymphoma patients, of whom 20 are known to have died

Survival time in months	Number of deaths	Number at risk	Estimated probability of survival	Standard error of estimate
2.5	1	31	0.968	0.032
4.1	1	30	0.935	0.044
4.6	1	29	0.903	0.053
6.4	1	28	0.871	0.060
6.7	1	27	0.839	0.066
7.4	1	26	0.806	0.071
7.6	1	25	0.774	0.075
7.7	1	24	0.742	0.079
7.8	1	23	0.710	0.082
8.8	1	22	0.677	0.084
13.3	1	21	0.645	0.086
13.4	1	20	0.613	0.087
18.3	1	19	0.581	0.089
19.7	1	18	0.548	0.089
21.9	1	17	0.516	0.090
24.7	1	16	0.484	0.090
27.5	1	15	0.452	0.089
29.7	1	14	0.419	0.089
32.9	1	12	0.384	0.088
33.5	1	11	0.349	0.087

6.3. Computing the Kaplan-Meier Estimate

In this final section of chapter 6 we intend to discuss, in some detail, a simple method for calculating the Kaplan-Meier estimate by hand. The technique is not complicated; nevertheless, some readers may prefer to omit this section and proceed to chapter 7, where we consider a method for comparing the survival experience of two or more groups of patients.

To calculate a Kaplan-Meier estimated survival curve, it is first necessary to list all observations, censored and uncensored, in increasing order. The convention is adopted that if both observed and censored survival times of the same duration have been recorded, then the uncensored observations precede the corresponding censored survival times in the ordered list. For the simple example presented in Figure 6.2a, the ordered list of observations, in days, is

1*, 3, 4*, 5, 5, 6*, 7, 7, 7*, 8*

where * indicates a censored survival time.

The second step in the calculation is to draw up a table with six columns labelled as follows:

t	observed distinct survival times, in days
r	the number of deaths recorded at t days
n	the number of individuals still under observation at t days
p_c	the proportion of individuals under observation at t days who do not die at t days, i.e., $(n - r)/n$
$\Pr(T > t)$	the estimated probability of survival beyond t days
s.e.	the approximate standard error for the estimated probability of survival beyond t days

For convenience, the initial row of the table may be completed by entering $t = 0$, $r = 0$, $n = $ number of individuals in the study, $p_c = 1$, $\Pr(T > t) = 1$ and s.e. = blank. This simply indicates that the estimated survival curve begins with $\Pr(T > 0) = 1$, i.e., the estimated probability of survival beyond Day 0 is one. The first observed survival time in the ordered list of observations is then identified, and the number of observations which exceed this observed survival time is recorded, along with the number of deaths occurring at this specific time. Notice that the number of individuals still under observation at t days is equal to the number of individuals in the study minus the total number of observation times, censored or uncensored, which were less than t days.

In our example, the first observed survival time is t = 3; therefore, the initial two rows of the table would now be:

t	r	n	p_c	$Pr(T > t)$	s.e.
0	0	10	1.0	1.0	–
3	1	9			

The column labelled p_c gives the estimated probability of surviving Day t for individuals alive at t days. This is $(n-r)/n$, and $Pr(T > t)$, the estimated probability of survival beyond t days, is the product of the value of p_c from the current line and the value of $Pr(T > t)$ from the preceding line of the table. In the second row of our example table then, $p_c = 8/9 = 0.89$ and $Pr(T > t) = 0.89 \times 1.0 = 0.89$. According to the formula given in comment (c) of §6.2 for an approximate standard error for $Pr(T > t)$, the entry in the s.e. column will be:

$$Pr(T > t) \sqrt{\{1 - Pr(T > t)\}/n} = 0.89 \sqrt{(1 - 0.89)/9} = 0.10.$$

This process is then repeated for the next observed survival time. According to the ordered list for our example, r = 2 deaths are recorded at t = 5, at which time n = 7 individuals are still under observation. Therefore, $p_c = (7-2)/7 = 0.71$, $Pr(T > t) = 0.71 \times 0.89 = 0.64$, and s.e. $= 0.64\sqrt{0.36/7} = 0.15$. The table now looks like the following:

t	r	n	p_c	$Pr(T > t)$	s.e.
0	0	10	1.0	1.0	–
3	1	9	0.89	0.89	0.10
5	2	7	0.71	0.64	0.15

The final row in the table will correspond to the r = 2 deaths which are recorded at t = 7, when n = 4 individuals are still under observation. In this row, therefore, $p_c = 2/4 = 0.50$, $Pr(T > t) = 0.64 \times 0.50 = 0.32$ and s.e. $= 0.32\sqrt{0.68/4} = 0.13$. Thus, the completed table for our simple example is:

t	r	n	p_c	Pr(T > t)	s.e.
0	0	10	1.0	1.0	–
3	1	9	0.89	0.89	0.10
5	2	7	0.71	0.64	0.15
7	2	4	0.50	0.32	0.13

To plot the K-M estimated survival curve from the completed table, use the values in columns one and five (labelled t and Pr(T > t)) to draw the graph with its characteristic staircase appearance. Steps will occur at the values of the distinct observed survival times, i.e., the values of t. To the right of each value of t, draw a horizontal section at a height equal to the corresponding value of Pr(T > t). Each horizontal section will extend from the current value of t to the next value of t, where the next decrease in the graph occurs.

From the columns labelled t and Pr(T > t) in the table for our example, we see that the graph of the K-M estimated survival curve has a horizontal section from t = 0 to t = 3 at probability 1.0, a horizontal section from t = 3 to t = 5 at probability 0.89, a horizontal section from t = 5 to t = 7 at probability 0.64, and a horizontal section from t = 7 at probability 0.32. Since the final entry in the table for Pr(T > t) is not zero, the last horizontal section of the graph is terminated at the largest censored survival time in the ordered list of observations, namely 8. Therefore, the final horizontal section of the graph at probability 0.32 extends from t = 7 to t = 8; the estimated probability of survival is not defined for t > 8 in this particular case.

If the final censored observation, 8, had been an observed survival time instead, then the completed table would have been:

t	r	n	p_c	Pr(T > t)	s.e.
0	0	0	1.0	1.0	–
3	1	9	0.89	0.89	0.10
5	2	7	0.71	0.64	0.15
7	2	4	0.50	0.32	0.13
8	1	1	0.00	0.00	–

In this case, the graph of the K-M estimated survival curve would drop to zero at t = 8 and be equal to zero thereafter.

In general, the K-M estimated survival curve is used merely as a pictorial representation of the observed survival experience. It is common, however, to want to compare the survival experience of two or more groups of patients. Although standard errors can be used for this purpose, better techniques are available. These include the log-rank test, which we describe in chapter 7.

7 The Log-Rank or Mantel-Haenszel Test for the Comparison of Survival Curves

7.1. Introduction

In medical research, we frequently wish to compare the survival (or relapse, etc.) experience of two groups of individuals. The groups will differ with respect to a certain factor (treatment, age, sex, stage of disease, etc.), and it is the effect of this factor on survival which is of interest. For example, Figure 7.1 presents the Kaplan-Meier estimated survival curves for the 31 lymphoma patients mentioned in chapter 6, and a second group of 33 lymphoma patients who were diagnosed without clinical symptoms. According to standard practice, the 31 patients with clinical symptoms are said to have 'B' symptoms, while the other 33 have 'A' symptoms. Figure 7.1 shows an apparent survival advantage for patients with A symptoms.

In the discussion that follows, we present a test of the null hypothesis that the survival functions for patients with A and B symptoms are the same, even though their respective Kaplan-Meier estimates, which are based on random samples from the two populations, will inevitably differ. This test, which is called the log-rank or Mantel-Haenszel test, is only one of many tests which could be devised; nevertheless, it is frequently used to compare the survival functions of two or more populations.

The log-rank test is designed particularly to detect a difference between survival curves which results when the mortality rate in one group is consistently higher than the corresponding rate in a second group and the ratio of these two rates is constant over time. This is equivalent to saying that, provided an individual has survived for t units, the chance of dying in a brief interval following t is k times greater in one group than in the other, and the same statement is true for all values of t. The null hypothesis that there is no difference in survival experience between the two groups is represented by the value $k = 1$, i.e., a ratio of one. As we indicated in chapter 6, time is usually measured from some well-defined event such as diagnosis.

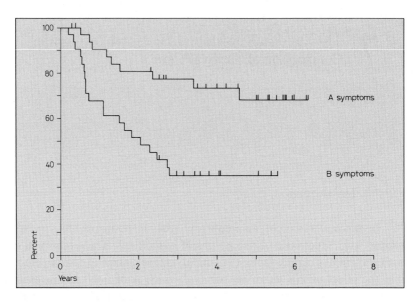

Fig. 7.1. The Kaplan-Meier estimated survival curves for 33 lymphoma patients presenting with A symptoms and 31 with B symptoms.

7.2. Details of the Test

The basic idea underlying the log-rank test involves examining each occasion when one or more deaths (or events) occurs. Based on the number of individuals in each group who are alive just before the observed death time and the total number of deaths observed at that time, we can calculate how many deaths would be expected in each group if the null hypothesis is true, i.e., if the mortality rates are identical. For example, if Group 1 has six individuals alive at t units and Group 2 has three, then the observed deaths at t should be distributed in the ratio 2:1 between the two groups, if the null hypothesis is true. If three deaths actually occurred at t units, then we would expect two in the first group and one in the second group. If only one death had actually occurred at t, then we would say that the expected number of deaths in Group 1 is 2/3 and in Group 2 is 1/3. Notice that the expected number of deaths need not correspond to a positive integer.

To complete the log-rank test we add up, for the two groups separately, the observed and expected numbers of deaths at all observed death times. These numbers are then compared. If O_1 and O_2 are the observed numbers of deaths in the two groups and E_1 and E_2 are the expected numbers of deaths calculated by summing the expected numbers at each event time, then the statistic used for comparison purposes is

$$T = \frac{(O_1 - E_1)^2}{E_1} + \frac{(O_2 - E_2)^2}{E_2}.$$

If the null hypothesis is true, T should be distributed approximately as a χ_1^2 random variable (chi-squared with one degree of freedom). Let t_0 represent the observed value of T for a particular set of data; then the significance level of the log-rank test is given by $Pr(T \geq t_0)$, which is approximately equal to $Pr(\chi_1^2 \geq t_0)$. Therefore, we can use Table 4.10 to evaluate the significance level of the log-rank test (see §4.4).

Comments:

(a) If we wish to compare the survival experience in two groups specified, say, by treatment, but it is important to adjust the comparison for another prognostic factor, say stage of the disease, then a stratified log-rank test may be performed. In this case, study subjects must be classified into strata according to stage, and within each stratum the calculations of observed and expected numbers of deaths for a log-rank test are performed. The test statistic, T, is computed from values of O_1, O_2, E_1 and E_2 which are obtained by summing the corresponding observed and expected values from all the strata.

The effectiveness of stratification as a means of adjusting for other prognostic factors is limited because it is necessary, simultaneously, to retain a moderate number of subjects in each stratum. If we wish to adjust for a number of prognostic factors then, in principle, we can define prognostic strata within which prognosis would be similar, except for the effect of treatment. However, as the number of prognostic factors increases, the strata soon become too small to be meaningful. Unless the study is very large, the use of more than six or eight strata is generally unwise. Stratification is probably most effective with two to four strata, especially since there are procedures which are more useful when the number of prognostic factors is large. These procedures will be discussed in chapter 12.

(b) It is possible to restrict the comparison of survival experience in two groups to a specified interval of the observation period, since the log-rank test is still valid when it is restricted in this way. However, it is important not to choose such restricted time intervals by examining the observed data and selecting an interval where the mortality looks different; this method of choosing an interval invalidates the calculation of the p-value because it constitutes selective sampling from the observed survival experience. On the other hand, it would be very reasonable to examine, separately, early and late mortality in the two treatment groups, if the time periods early and late are defined in some natural way.

(c) The log-rank test is always a valid test of the null hypothesis that the survival functions of two populations are the same. The effectiveness of the test in detecting departures from this hypothesis does depend on the form of the difference. The log-rank test is, in some sense, optimal if the difference arises because the mortality rate in one group is a constant multiple of the corresponding rate in the other group. If this is not the case, then the log-rank test may not be able to detect a difference that does exist. The importance of this assumption that there is a constant difference in mortality across time is another reason for performing the log-rank test on suitably-defined, restricted time intervals; doing so helps to validate the constant difference assumption for the data at hand.

(d) There are a number of alternative tests for comparing the survival experience of two groups. We do not intend to discuss these tests except to mention, briefly, another commonly-used test called the generalized Wilcoxon test. The latter differs from the log-rank test in that it attaches more importance to early deaths than to later deaths, whereas the log-rank test gives equal weight to all deaths. Thus, differences in the early survival experience of two populations are more likely to be detected by the generalized Wilcoxon test than by the log-rank test which we have described.

If survival data include censored observations, then there are different versions of the generalized Wilcoxon test which may be used. Although the details of their research are beyond the scope of this book, the work of *Prentice and Marek* [1979] suggests that *Gehan's* [1965] generalization is subject to serious criticism and probably should be avoided. An alternative, called *Peto's* generalized Wilcoxon statistic [see *Peto and Peto,* 1972], is preferable in this case.

(e) The use of $T = \frac{(O_1 - E_1)^2}{E_1} + \frac{(O_2 - E_2)^2}{E_2}$ as the test statistic, and the assumption that T has a χ_1^2 distribution if the null hypothesis is true, is an approximation which is particularly convenient for hand calculations. This approximation can be improved and, frequently, computer programs to calculate the log-rank test will use an alternative form of the statistic. We will not discuss any of these improved versions, except to note that the principle and nature of the test are unchanged.

(f) The log-rank test can be generalized to test for the equality of survival experience in more than two study populations (groups). The total number of deaths at each event time, and the proportions of the study subjects in each group at that time, are used to calculate the expected numbers of deaths in each group if the null hypothesis is true. The totals O and E are calculated for each group, and the test statistic, T, is the sum of the quantity $(O - E)^2/E$ for each group. If the null hypothesis is true, T is distributed approximately as a χ^2_{k-1} variable (chi-squared with k–1 degrees of freedom), where k is the number of groups whose survival experience is being compared.

7.3. Evaluating the Log-Rank Test - A Simple Example

Although statisticians will frequently use a computer to evaluate the log-rank test for a given set of data, the actual calculations are not particularly complicated. To illustrate exactly what is involved, we consider the simple example shown in Table 7.1. This table presents two sets of survival times; those in Group 1 correspond to the times used in the example discussed in §6.3. To perform the calculations required for a log-rank test, it is convenient to set up a table with ten columns. The column headings will be the following:

t	the event time, in days
n	the number of individuals still under observation at t days
n_1	the number of individuals in Group 1 still under observation at t days
n_2	the number of individuals in Group 2 still under observation at t days
r	the number of deaths recorded at t days
c	the number of censored values recorded at t days
o_1	the number of deaths in Group 1 recorded at t days
o_2	the number of deaths in Group 2 recorded at t days
e_1	the expected number of deaths in Group 1 at t days
e_2	the expected number of deaths in Group 2 at t days

Chronologically, the first event recorded in Table 7.1 is a censored value occurring at t = 1. Although this event actually contributes nothing to our test statistic, it is convenient, for completeness, to include a row in the table for this censored value. The event time is t = 1, the total number of observations is n = 18, of which $n_1 = 10$ and $n_2 = 8$ are in Groups 1 and 2, respectively. At

Table 7.1. Hypothetical survival times, in days, for the comparison of mortality in two groups; a * indicates a censored observation

Group 1	1*, 3, 4*, 5, 5, 6*, 7, 7, 7*, 8
Group 2	2, 2, 3*, 4, 6*, 6*, 7, 10

$t = 1$ there are $r = 0$ deaths and $c = 1$ censored values. Since no deaths were observed, the observed and expected numbers of deaths are all zero as well. Therefore, the first row of the table is:

t	n	n_1	n_2	r	c	o_1	o_2	e_1	e_2
1	18	10	8	0	1	0	0	0	0

The second event time in our hypothetical study is $t = 2$, at which two deaths were recorded in Group 2. One observation was censored at $t = 1$; therefore, at $t = 2$ we have $n = 17$ individuals under observation, of which $n_1 = 9$ and $n_2 = 8$ are in Groups 1 and 2, respectively. The number of deaths is $r = 2$ and the number of censored observations is $c = 0$. The observed numbers of deaths are $o_1 = 0$ in Group 1 and $o_2 = 2$ in Group 2. The proportion of individuals under observation in Group 1 is $\frac{9}{17}$ and in Group 2 it is $\frac{8}{17}$. Therefore, the expected numbers of deaths in the two groups, given that there were two observed deaths, are $e_1 = 2 \times \frac{9}{17} = 1.06$ and $e_2 = 2 \times \frac{8}{17} = 0.94$. Notice that, except for rounding errors in the calculations, it should be true that $r = o_1 + o_2 = e_1 + e_2$. With the second row completed the table now becomes

t	n	n_1	n_2	r	c	o_1	o_2	e_1	e_2
1	18	10	8	0	1	0	0	0	0
2	17	9	8	2	0	0	2	1.06	0.94

At the third event time, $t = 3$, there is one death recorded in Group 1 and one censored observation in Group 2. At $t = 3$ there were $n = 15$ individuals still under observation, of which $n_1 = 9$ and $n_2 = 6$ were in Groups 1 and 2, respectively. Notice that, in each row of the table, the current value of n is the value of n from the preceding row minus the sum of r and c from the preceding row. At $t = 3$ there was $r = 1$ death and $c = 1$ censored value with $o_1 = 1$ and $o_2 = 0$; therefore, the expected numbers of deaths are $e_1 = 1 \times \frac{9}{15} = 0.60$ and $e_2 = 1 \times \frac{6}{15} = 0.40$.

Additional rows are added to the table until the last observed death is recorded, or until n_1 or n_2 becomes zero. The completed table for the example is given in Figure 7.2.

Column Headings

t	the event time, in days
n	the number of individuals still under observation at t days
n_1	the number of individuals in Group 1 still under observation at t days
n_2	the number of individuals in Group 2 still under observation at t days
r	the number of deaths recorded at t days
c	the number of censored values recorded at t days
o_1	the number of deaths in Group 1 recorded at t days
o_2	the number of deaths in Group 2 recorded at t days
e_1	the expected number of deaths in Group 1 at t days
e_2	the expected number of deaths in Group 2 at t days

t	n	n_1	n_2	r	c	o_1	o_2	$e_1 = \dfrac{r \times n_1}{n}$	$e_2 = \dfrac{r \times n_2}{n}$
1	18	10	8	0	1	0	0	$\dfrac{0 \times 10}{18} = 0.00$	$\dfrac{0 \times 8}{18} = 0.00$
2	17	9	8	2	0	0	2	$\dfrac{2 \times 9}{17} = 1.06$	$\dfrac{2 \times 8}{17} = 0.94$
3	15	9	6	1	1	1	0	$\dfrac{1 \times 9}{15} = 0.60$	$\dfrac{1 \times 6}{15} = 0.40$
4	13	8	5	1	1	0	1	$\dfrac{1 \times 8}{13} = 0.62$	$\dfrac{1 \times 5}{13} = 0.38$
5	11	7	4	2	0	2	0	$\dfrac{2 \times 7}{11} = 1.27$	$\dfrac{2 \times 4}{11} = 0.73$
6	9	5	4	0	3	0	0	$\dfrac{0 \times 5}{9} = 0.00$	$\dfrac{0 \times 4}{9} = 0.00$
7	6	4	2	3	1	2	1	$\dfrac{3 \times 4}{6} = 2.00$	$\dfrac{3 \times 2}{6} = 1.00$
8	2	1	1	1	0	1	0	$\dfrac{1 \times 1}{2} = 0.50$	$\dfrac{1 \times 1}{2} = 0.50$
Totals						6	4	6.05	3.95

$$t_o = \frac{(6 - 6.05)^2}{6.05} + \frac{(4 - 3.95)^2}{3.95} = 0.001$$

Fig. 7.2. Details of the log-rank test calculations for the data presented in Table 7.1.

When the table has been completed, the last four columns must be summed to obtain $O_1 = \Sigma\, o_1 = 6$, $O_2 = \Sigma\, o_2 = 4$, $E_1 = \Sigma\, e_1 = 6.05$ and $E_2 = \Sigma\, e_2 = 3.95$. Since the observed value of T, which is calculated in Figure 7.2, is $t_o = 0.001$, the significance level of the data with respect to the null hypothesis is given by $Pr(\chi_1^2 \geqslant 0.001)$. According to Table 4.10, $Pr(\chi_1^2 \geqslant 0.001) > 0.25$. Therefore, we conclude that the data provide no evidence to contradict the null hypothesis that the survival functions for Groups 1 and 2 are the same.

7.4. A More Realistic Example

Table 7.2 presents the data for the two Kaplan-Meier estimated survival curves shown in Figure 7.1. The observed numbers of deaths in the A and B symptoms groups were 9 and 20, respectively. The log-rank calculations lead to corresponding expected numbers of deaths of 17.07 and 11.93. Therefore, the observed value of the log-rank test statistic for these data is

$$t_o = \frac{(9-17.07)^2}{17.07} + \frac{(20-11.93)^2}{11.93} = 9.275.$$

If the null hypothesis of no difference in survival experience between the two groups is true, t_o should be an observation from a χ_1^2 distribution. Therefore, the significance level of the data is equal to

$$Pr(\chi_1^2 \geqslant 9.275) = 0.0023.$$

Using Table 4.10, we can only determine that $0.005 > Pr(\chi_1^2 \geqslant 9.275) > 0.001$; the exact value was obtained from other sources. In either case, we would conclude that the data do provide evidence against the null hypothesis and suggest that lymphoma patients with A symptoms enjoy a real survival advantage.

Notice that the essence of the test is to conclude that we have evidence contradicting the null hypothesis when the observed numbers of deaths in the two groups are significantly different from the corresponding numbers which would be expected, if the survival functions for the two groups of patients are the same.

In subsequent chapters, we intend to present important extensions and generalizations of the methods we have already discussed. However, we first need to introduce certain notions and concepts which are based on the normal, or Gaussian, distribution. In general, statistical methods for normal data

Table 7.2. Survival times, in months, for 64 lymphoma patients; a * indicates a censored survival time

A symptoms	3.2*, 4.4*, 6.2, 9.0, 9.9, 14.4, 15.8, 18.5, 27.6*, 28.5, 30.1*, 31.5*, 32.2*, 41.0, 41.8*, 44.5*, 47.8*, 50.6*, 54.3*, 55.0, 60.0*, 60.4*, 63.6*, 63.7*, 63.8*, 66.1*, 68.0*, 68.7*, 68.8*, 70.9*, 71.5*, 75.3*, 75.7*
B symptoms	2.5, 4.1, 4.6, 6.4, 6.7, 7.4, 7.6, 7.7, 7.8, 8.8, 13.3, 13.4, 18.3, 19.7, 21.9, 24.7, 27.5, 29.7, 30.1*, 32.9, 33.5, 35.4*, 37.7*, 40.9*, 42.6*, 45.4*, 48.5*, 48.9*, 60.4*, 64.4*, 66.4*

comprise a major fraction of the material presented in elementary textbooks on statistics. Although the role of this methodology is not as prominent in research into chronic diseases, the techniques still represent an important set of basic, investigative tools for both the statistician and the medical researcher. In addition, the normal distribution plays a rather important part in much of the advanced methodology that we intend to discuss in chapters 10 to 12. Therefore, in chapter 8, we will introduce the normal distribution from that perspective. Chapter 9 contains details of the specific methods which can be used with data which are assumed to be normally distributed.

8 An Introduction to the Normal Distribution

8.1. Introduction

In chapter 1, the normal distribution was used to describe the variation in systolic blood pressure. In most introductory books on statistics, and even in many advanced texts, the normal probability distribution is prominent. By comparison, in the first seven chapters of this book the normal distribution has been mentioned only once. This shift in emphasis has occurred because the specific test procedures which are appropriate for data from a normal distribution are not used as frequently in clinical research as they are in other settings such as the physical sciences or engineering. In fact, the nature of medical data often precludes the use of much of the methodology which assumes that the data are normally distributed. Nevertheless, there are certain situations where these techniques will be useful, and in chapter 9 we discuss a number of the specialized procedures which can be used to analyze normally distributed data.

There is another way that the normal distribution arises in medical statistics however, and for this reason, alone, it is essential to understand the basic theory of the normal distribution. Many of the advanced statistical methods that are being used in medical research today involve test statistics which have approximate normal distributions. This statement applies particularly to the methods which we intend to discuss in chapters 10, 11 and 12. Therefore, in the remainder of this chapter, we shall introduce the normal distribution. We have not previously discussed any probability distribution in quite as much detail as our scrutiny of the normal distribution will involve. Therefore, readers may find it helpful to know that a complete appreciation of §8.2 is not essential. The most important material concerns aspects of the normal distribution which are pertinent to its use in advanced methodology, and these topics are discussed in §§8.3, 8.4. However, §8.2 should be read before proceeding to the rest of the chapter.

8.2. Basic Features of the Normal Distribution

The normal distribution is used to describe a particular pattern of variation for a continuous random variable. Our discussion of continuous random variables in §1.2 emphasized the area = probability equation and introduced the cumulative probability curve as a means of calculating $\Pr(X \leqslant a)$, the probability that the random variable X is at most a. Equivalently, $\Pr(X \leqslant a)$ is the area under the probability curve for X which lies to the left of the vertical line at a.

Figure 8.1a shows the cumulative probability curve for a continuous random variable, Z, which has a *standardized* normal distribution. The upper case Roman letter Z is generally used to represent the standardized normal variable, and we will follow this convention in the remainder of the book.

The cumulative probability curve is very useful for calculating probabilities; however, the graph in Figure 8.1a does not convey particularly well the nature of the variation described by the standardized normal distribution. To appreciate this aspect of Z we need to examine its probability curve, shown in Figure 8.1b. Recall that the probability curve is the analogue of a histogram for a continuous random variable. Immediately we see that the standard normal distribution has a characteristic bell-like shape and is symmetric about the mean value, zero. Because of this symmetry about zero, it follows that for any positive number a, the probability that Z exceeds a is equal to the probability that Z is less than $-a$, i.e., $\Pr(Z > a) = \Pr(Z < -a)$. This equality is indicated in Figure 8.1b by the two shaded areas of equal size which represent these two probabilities.

In chapter 1, we described the mean, $E(X) = \mu$, and the variance, $\text{Var}(X) = \sigma^2$, as useful summary characteristics of a probability distribution. For the standardized normal distribution the mean is zero and the variance is one; that is, $\mu = 0$ and $\sigma^2 = 1$. These are, in fact, the particular characteristics which define the standardized normal distribution. Now, compare Figures 8.1a and 8.2a. Figure 8.2a shows the cumulative probability curve for a random variable, X, which is also normally distributed but which has mean μ and variance σ^2, i.e., $E(X) = \mu$, $\text{Var}(X) = \sigma^2$. The curve for X corresponds exactly with the cumulative probability curve for Z, shown in Figure 8.1a, except that the center of the horizontal axis in Figure 8.2a is μ rather than zero, and each major division on this axis represents one standard deviation, σ, rather than one unit. Clearly, if $\mu = 0$ and $\sigma = 1$, then X and Z would have identical cumulative probability curves. This is why the two values $E(Z) = 0$ and

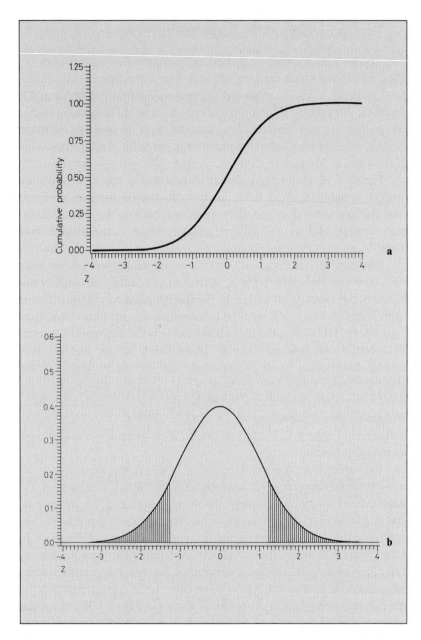

Fig. 8.1. The standardized normal distribution. **a** Cumulative probability curve. **b** Corresponding probability curve with shaded areas representing Pr(Z > a) and Pr(Z < −a).

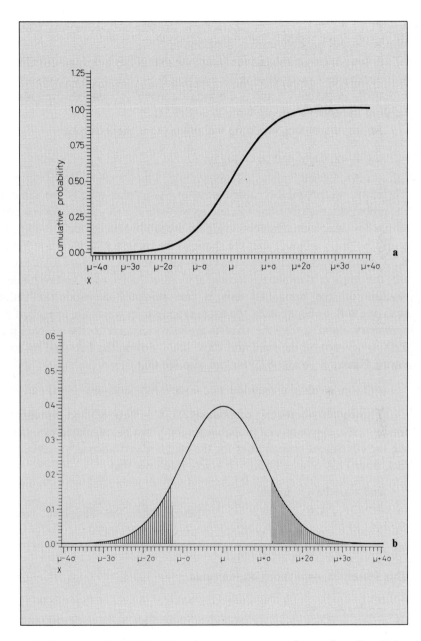

Fig. 8.2. The normal distribution with mean μ and variance σ². **a** Cumulative probability curve. **b** Corresponding probability curve with shaded areas representing $Pr(X > \mu + a\sigma)$ and $Pr(X < \mu - a\sigma)$.

Var(Z) = 1, i.e., $\mu = 0$, $\sigma^2 = 1$, characterize the standardized normal distribution among all possible normal distributions.

A convenient shorthand for specifying that X has a normal distribution with mean μ and variance σ^2 is the notation $X \sim N(\mu, \sigma^2)$, which we will use repeatedly in chapters 8 and 9. To indicate that Z is a standardized normal random variable we simply write $Z \sim N(0, 1)$.

An important fact which we will often use is the following:

$$\text{if } X \sim N(\mu, \sigma^2), \text{ then } \frac{X-\mu}{\sigma} \sim N(0, 1).$$

Therefore, the probability distribution of $(X-\mu)/\sigma$ is exactly the same as the probability distribution of Z, and so we write $Z = (X-\mu)/\sigma$. This relationship is best appreciated by comparing the probability curves for $X \sim N(\mu, \sigma^2)$ and $Z \sim N(0, 1)$. Notice that the shape of the curve for X, shown in Figure 8.2b, corresponds exactly with the curve for Z shown in Figure 8.1b, except that the center of symmetry is located at μ rather than at zero, and each major division on the horizontal axis is one standard deviation, σ, rather than one unit. In Figure 8.2b, the equal probabilities which are a result of the symmetry about μ (see the shaded areas) correspond to the probabilities $\Pr(X > \mu + a\sigma)$ on the right and $\Pr(X < \mu - a\sigma)$ on the left. And by comparing Figures 8.1b and 8.2b we can also see that

$$\Pr(Z > a) = \Pr(X > \mu + a\sigma) \text{ and } \Pr(Z < -a) = \Pr(X < \mu - a\sigma).$$

This equality between probabilities for $X \sim N(\mu, \sigma^2)$ and probabilities for $Z \sim N(0, 1)$ means that probabilities for X can be calculated by evaluating the equivalent probabilities for the standardized normal variable Z. In fact, since $\Pr(Z > a) = \Pr(X > \mu + a\sigma)$, it follows that

$$\Pr(Z > a) = \Pr(X > \mu + a\sigma)$$

$$= \Pr(X-\mu > a\sigma) \qquad \text{[subtract } \mu \text{ from both sides of the inequality]}$$

$$= \Pr\left(\frac{X-\mu}{\sigma} > a\right). \qquad \text{[divide both sides of the inequality by } \sigma\text{]}$$

This illustrates, once more, the fact that

$$\frac{X - \mu}{\sigma} = Z \sim N(0, 1) ,$$

i.e., the random variable $\frac{X-\mu}{\sigma}$ has a standardized normal distribution. This relationship, $Z = \frac{X-\mu}{\sigma}$, is usually called the standardizing transformation because it links the distribution of $X \sim N(\mu, \sigma^2)$ to the distribution of $Z \sim$

N(0, 1). In fact, the concept of the standardizing transformation is fundamental to the calculation of normal probabilities and to the use of the normal distribution in the advanced methodology we intend to discuss in chapters 10 through 12.

In §8.1, we indicated that the nature of medical data often precludes the use of methods which assume that the observations, e.g., survival times, are normally distributed. Why, then, is the normal distribution so important? A complete answer to this question goes well beyond the scope of our discussion. However, in general terms we can state that, according to a certain theorem in mathematical statistics called the central limit theorem, the probability distribution of the sum of observations from any population corresponds more and more to that of a normal distribution as the number of observations increases, i.e., if the sample size is large enough, the sum of observations from any distribution is approximately normally distributed. Since many of the test statistics and estimating functions which are used in advanced statistical methods can be represented as just such a sum, it follows that their approximate normal distributions can be used to calculate probabilities when nothing more exact is possible.

To counteract the solemn tone of the preceding explanation, and also to summarize our discussion of the basic features of the normal distribution, we conclude with a more light-hearted portrait of the normal probability curve which was devised by *W.J. Youden:*

THE

NORMAL

LAW OF ERROR

STANDS OUT IN THE

EXPERIENCE OF MANKIND

AS ONE OF THE BROADEST

GENERALIZATIONS OF NATURAL

PHILOSOPHY ♦ IT SERVES AS THE

GUIDING INSTRUMENT IN RESEARCHES

IN THE PHYSICAL AND SOCIAL SCIENCES AND

IN MEDICINE AGRICULTURE AND ENGINEERING ♦

IT IS AN INDISPENSABLE TOOL FOR THE ANALYSIS AND THE

INTERPRETATION OF THE BASIC DATA OBTAINED BY OBSERVATION AND EXPERIMENT

8.3. The Normal Distribution and Significance Testing

In this section and the next, we will focus attention on the role of the normal distribution in the more advanced statistical methods which we intend to introduce in chapters 10, 11 and 12.

Recall the survival data for 64 patients with lymphoma which were discussed in §7.4. In chapter 7, we used a log-rank test to study the possible survival advantage that patients presenting with A symptoms might enjoy relative to those who present with B symptoms. Since the significance level of the log-rank test was 0.0023, we concluded that the data provide evidence against the hypothesis of comparable survival in the two groups.

In chapter 12, we discuss a method for estimating the ratio of the separate mortality rates for patients presenting with A and B symptoms. This method leads to an estimate that the mortality rate for patients with B symptoms is 3.0 times that of patients with A symptoms. The actual calculations which are involved concern the logarithm of this ratio of mortality rates, which we represent by b, and lead to an estimate of b which we denote by $\hat{b} = \log 3.0 = 1.10$. Simultaneously, the calculations also yield $\hat{\sigma}$, the estimated standard deviation of $\hat{b}$; the value of $\hat{\sigma}$ is 0.41. The symbol $\hat{\ }$ indicates that $\hat{b}$ is an estimate of b and $\hat{\sigma}$ is an estimate of the standard deviation of $\hat{b}$. We will also use the phrase est. standard error ($\hat{b}$) interchangeably with $\hat{\sigma}$.

Much of the methodology in chapters 10, 11 and 12 is concerned with quantities like b. The usual question of interest is whether or not b equals zero, since this value frequently represents a lack of association between two variables of interest in a study. For example, in the lymphoma data, the value b = 0 corresponds to a ratio of mortality rates which is equal to $e^0 = 1.0$. Thus, b = 0 represents the hypothesis that there is no relationship between presenting symptoms and survival. In this section, we will consider a test of the hypothesis H: b = 0 which is based on the quantities $\hat{b}$ and $\hat{\sigma}$.

Because of the central limit theorem, which we discussed briefly at the end of §8.2, we can state that $\hat{b}$, which is usually a complicated function of the data, has an approximate normal distribution with mean b and variance $\hat{\sigma}^2$, i.e., $\hat{b} \sim N(b, \hat{\sigma}^2)$. We can remark here, without any attempt at justification, that one reason for using the logarithm of the ratio of mortality rates, rather than the ratio itself, is that the logarithmic transformation generally improves the accuracy of the normal approximation. Since $\hat{b} \sim N(b, \hat{\sigma}^2)$, to test H: b = 0 we assume that $\hat{b} \sim N(0, \hat{\sigma}^2)$, i.e., assume that the hypothesis is true,

Table 8.1. Critical values of the probability distribution of T = |Z|; the table specifies values of the number t_0 such that $Pr(T \geqslant t_0) = p$

	Probability level, p				
	0.10	0.05	0.01	0.005	0.001
t_0	1.645	1.960	2.576	2.807	3.291

and evaluate the degree to which an observed value of $\hat{b}$, say b_0, is consistent with this particular normal distribution. If $\hat{b} \sim N(0, \hat{\sigma}^2)$, then the standardizing transformation ensures that

$$Z = \frac{\hat{b}-0}{\hat{\sigma}} = \frac{\hat{b}}{\hat{\sigma}} \sim N(0, 1).$$

In general, both positive and negative values of $\hat{b}$ can constitute evidence against the hypothesis that b is zero. This prompts us to use the normal test statistic

$$T = \frac{|\hat{b}|}{\hat{\sigma}} = \frac{|\hat{b}|}{\text{est. standard error } (\hat{b})},$$

to test H: b = 0; recall that $|\hat{b}|$ means that we should change the sign of $\hat{b}$ if its value is negative. Let t_0 be the observed value of T which corresponds to b_0, i.e., $t_0 = |b_0|/\hat{\sigma}$. Since T is always non-negative, values which exceed t_0 are less consistent with the null hypothesis than the observed data. Therefore, the significance level of the test is $Pr(T \geqslant t_0)$, which is equal to $Pr(|Z| \geqslant t_0)$ since T = |Z|.

Although $Pr(T \geqslant t_0)$ can be calculated exactly, it is more common in the medical literature to compare t_0 with selected critical values for the distribution of T. These can be derived from the cumulative probability curve for Z, and are tabulated in Table 8.1. This use of critical values for the probability distribution of T in order to determine the significance level of the data corresponds exactly with our use of statistical tables for the χ^2 distribution in chapters 4, 5 and 7.

Although the distinction between the random variable $\hat{b}$ and its observed value b_0 is technically correct, this difference is often not maintained in practice. As we have indicated earlier, the results in the case of the lymphoma data would be summarized as $\hat{b} = 1.10$ and $\hat{\sigma} = 0.41$. Therefore, the observed value of the test statistic, which is often called a normal deviate, is

$$\frac{\hat{b}}{\hat{\sigma}} = \frac{1.10}{0.41} = 2.68,$$

and by referring to Table 8.1 we can see that the significance level of the lymphoma data with respect to the hypothesis $b = 0$ is between 0.01 and 0.005, i.e., $0.005 < p < 0.01$. This indicates that the data provide strong evidence against the null hypothesis that b equals zero, i.e., against the hypothesis of identical survival experience in the two patient groups. We reached the same conclusion in §7.4 after using a log-rank test to analyze the survival times.

In §8.5, we describe how tables of the standardized normal distribution can be used to calculate p-values more precisely. At this point, however, it seems appropriate to indicate the link between the χ_1^2 distribution, which was prominent in previous chapters, and the probability distributions of Z and $T = |Z|$. It can be shown that $T^2 = Z^2 \sim \chi_1^2$; therefore,

$$\Pr(T \geqslant t_0) = \Pr(T^2 \geqslant t_0^2) = \Pr(Z^2 \geqslant t_0^2) = \Pr(\chi_1^2 \geqslant t_0^2).$$

This equation specifies that statistical tables for the χ_1^2 distribution can also be used to evaluate the significance level of an observed Z-statistic, i.e., an observed value of T. To use the χ_1^2 table, we first need to square t_0. Occasionally, this relationship between T and the χ_1^2 distribution is used to present the results of an analysis. In general, however, significance levels are calculated from observed Z-statistics by referring to critical values for the distribution of $T = |Z|$, cf., Table 8.1.

8.4. The Normal Distribution and Confidence Intervals

In all the statistical methods which we have thus far considered, the use of significance tests as a means of interpreting data has been emphasized. The concept of statistical estimation was introduced in chapter 6, but has otherwise been absent from our discussion. Although significance tests predominate in the medical literature, we can discern a slight shift towards the greater use of estimation procedures, the most useful of which incorporate the calculation of confidence intervals. From the statistical point of view, this is a development which is long overdue.

The perspective which we intend to adopt in this section is a narrow one; a definitive exposition of the topic of confidence intervals goes beyond the purpose of this book. There are well-defined methods for calculating confidence intervals in all of the situations that we have previously described; we shall not consider any of these techniques, although the calculations are generally not difficult. In chapter 9, we will introduce the calculation of a confidence interval for the mean of a population when the data are normally distributed. This particular interval arises naturally in our discussion of specialized procedures for data of this kind. However, in this section we will consider only those confidence intervals which pertain to the role of the normal distribution in the advanced statistical methods which are the subject of chapters 10, 11 and 12. In this way, our discussion will parallel that of the preceding section.

In chapter 2, we defined a significance test to be a statistical procedure which determines the degree to which observed data are consistent with a specific hypothesis about a population. Frequently, the hypothesis concerns the value of a specific parameter which, in some sense, characterizes the population, e.g., μ or σ^2. By suitably revising the wording of this definition, we can accurately describe one method of obtaining confidence intervals. Basically, a confidence interval can be regarded as the result of a statistical procedure which identifies the set of all plausible values of a specific parameter. These will be values of the parameter which are consistent with the observed data. In fact, a confidence interval consists of every possible value of the parameter which, if tested as a specific null hypothesis in the usual way, would not lead us to conclude that the data contradict that particular null hypothesis.

Suppose, as in the previous section, that $\hat{b}$ is an estimate of a parameter b, generated by one of the methods described in chapters 10 through 12; we have stated that the distribution of $\hat{b}$ is approximately normal with mean b and variance $\hat{\sigma}^2$, i.e., $\hat{b} \sim N(b, \hat{\sigma}^2)$. Now imagine that we wish to test the hypothesis that b is equal to the specific value b_1, say. The appropriate test statistic is $T = |\hat{b} - b_1| / \hat{\sigma}$, and if the observed value of T which we obtain is less than 1.96 (cf., Table 8.1), then the corresponding significance level exceeds 0.05 since $Pr(T \geqslant 1.96) = 0.05$. Consequently, we would conclude that the value b_1 is plausible, since the hypothesis H: $b = b_1$ is not contradicted by the data ($p > 0.05$). Now if b_1 is the true value of b, we know that $Pr(T \leqslant 1.96) = 0.95$. But we can also interpret this probability statement in the following way: the probability that our interval of plausible values will include the specific value b_1 is 0.95, if b_1 is, in fact, the true value of b. For this reason, the interval of plausible values is called a 95% confidence interval; we are 95% sure, or confident, that the true value of b will be included in the interval of values which are consistent with the data.

To actually carry out a significance test for each possible value of b would be an enormous task. Fortunately, the actual calculations only need to be performed once, using algebraic symbols rather than actual numbers. This calculation determines that the set of all possible values of the parameter which are consistent with the data, i.e., $p > 0.05$, is the interval $(\hat{b} - 1.96\hat{\sigma}, \hat{b} + 1.96\hat{\sigma})$. Notice that this interval is completely determined by the data, which are summarized in the values of $\hat{b}$ and $\hat{\sigma}$, and by the value 1.96 from the normal distribution, corresponding to the 5% critical value which we use to judge consistency. Since we are 95% sure that this interval includes the true value of b, $(\hat{b} - 1.96\hat{\sigma}, \hat{b} + 1.96\hat{\sigma})$ is called a 95% confidence interval for b.

Although 95% confidence intervals are the most common, since they correspond to the familiar 5% significance level, there is no theoretical reason which prevents the use of other levels of confidence, for example, 90 or 99%. It should be clear that, if we want a 99% confidence interval for b instead of a 95% confidence interval, we are choosing to judge consistency on the basis of the 1% critical value for the distribution of T. According to Table 8.1, this number is 2.576. Therefore, if we replace 1.96, the 5% critical value, by 2.576, we will obtain $(\hat{b} - 2.576\hat{\sigma}, \hat{b} + 2.576\hat{\sigma})$, the 99% confidence interval for b. Or we could use $(\hat{b} - 1.645\hat{\sigma}, \hat{b} + 1.645\hat{\sigma})$, the 90% confidence interval for b.

From these formulae, we can make an important observation about the relationship between the length of the confidence interval and the level of confidence. The length of the 90% interval is $2(1.645)\hat{\sigma} = 3.29\hat{\sigma}$; the corresponding values for the 95 and 99% intervals are $3.92\hat{\sigma}$ and $5.152\hat{\sigma}$, respectively. Therefore, if we wish to increase our confidence that the interval includes the true value of b, the interval will necessarily be longer.

For the lymphoma data which we discussed in §8.3, we have stated that the method of chapter 12 leads to an estimate for b, the logarithm of the ratio of mortality rates, which is $\hat{b} = 1.10$; the estimated standard error of $\hat{b}$ is $\hat{\sigma} = 0.41$. Therefore, a 95% confidence interval for the true value of b is the set of values

$$\{1.10 - 1.96(0.41), 1.10 + 1.96(0.41)\} = (0.30, 1.90).$$

But what information is conveyed by this interval of values for b? In particular, does this 95% confidence interval provide information concerning the survival of lymphoma patients which we could not deduce from the significance test which was discussed in §8.3?

The test of significance prompted us to conclude that symptom classification does influence survival. Given this conclusion, a token examination of the data would indicate that the mortality rate is higher for those patients who present with B symptoms. Notice that this same information can also be deduced from the confidence interval. The value b = 0, which corresponds to equal survival experience in the two groups, is excluded from the 95% confidence interval for b; therefore, in light of the data, b = 0 is not a plausible value. Moreover, all values in the interval are positive, corresponding to a higher estimated mortality rate in the patients with B symptoms.

But there is additional practical information in the 95% confidence interval for b. The data generate an estimate of $\exp(\hat{b}) = 3.0$ for the ratio of the mortality rates. However, the width of the confidence interval for b characterizes the precision of this estimate. Although 3.0 is, in some sense, our best estimate of the ratio of the mortality rates, we know that the data are also consistent with a ratio as low as $\exp(0.30) = 1.35$, or as high as $\exp(1.90) = 6.69$. If knowledge that this ratio is at least as high as 1.35 is sufficient grounds to justify a change in treatment patterns, then such an alteration might be implemented. On the other hand, if a ratio of 2.0, for example, was necessary to justify the change, then the researchers would know that additional data were needed in order to make the estimation of b more precise. In general, a narrow confidence interval reflects the fact that we have fairly precise knowledge concerning the value of b, whereas a wide confidence interval indicates that our knowledge of b, and the effect it represents, is rather imprecise and therefore less informative.

In succeeding chapters, we will use significance tests, parameter estimates and confidence intervals to present the analyses of medical studies which demonstrate the use of more advanced statistical methodology. By emphasizing this combined approach to the analysis of data, we hope to make confidence intervals more attractive, and more familiar, to medical researchers.

It is probably true that most medical researchers will have little need to know more than the selected critical values presented in Table 8.1. Nevertheless, precise p-values are often quoted in the medical literature, and we will do the same in subsequent chapters. The next section describes how to use a table of the cumulative probability curve for the standardized normal distribution. The exposition is necessarily somewhat detailed. Therefore, readers who are willing to accept, on trust, a few precise p-values may safely omit §8.5 and proceed to chapter 9.

Table 8.2. Values of the cumulative probability function, $\Phi(z) = \Pr(Z \leqslant z)$, for the standardized normal distribution

z	0.00	0.01	0.02	0.03	0.04	0.05	0.06	0.07	0.08	0.09
0.0	0.5000	0.5040	0.5080	0.5120	0.5160	0.5199	0.5239	0.5279	0.5319	0.5359
0.1	0.5398	0.5438	0.5478	0.5517	0.5557	0.5596	0.5636	0.5675	0.5714	0.5753
0.2	0.5793	0.5832	0.5871	0.5910	0.5948	0.5987	0.6026	0.6064	0.6103	0.6141
0.3	0.6179	0.6217	0.6255	0.6293	0.6331	0.6368	0.6406	0.6443	0.6480	0.6517
0.4	0.6554	0.6591	0.6628	0.6664	0.6700	0.6736	0.6772	0.6808	0.6844	0.6879
0.5	0.6915	0.6950	0.6985	0.7019	0.7054	0.7088	0.7123	0.7157	0.7190	0.7224
0.6	0.7257	0.7291	0.7324	0.7357	0.7389	0.7422	0.7454	0.7486	0.7517	0.7549
0.7	0.7580	0.7611	0.7642	0.7673	0.7704	0.7734	0.7764	0.7794	0.7823	0.7852
0.8	0.7881	0.7910	0.7939	0.7967	0.7995	0.8023	0.8051	0.8078	0.8106	0.8133
0.9	0.8159	0.8186	0.8212	0.8238	0.8264	0.8289	0.8315	0.8340	0.8365	0.8389
1.0	0.8413	0.8438	0.8461	0.8485	0.8508	0.8531	0.8554	0.8577	0.8599	0.8621
1.1	0.8643	0.8665	0.8686	0.8708	0.8729	0.8749	0.8770	0.8790	0.8810	0.8830
1.2	0.8849	0.8869	0.8888	0.8907	0.8925	0.8944	0.8962	0.8980	0.8997	0.9015
1.3	0.9032	0.9049	0.9066	0.9082	0.9099	0.9115	0.9131	0.9147	0.9162	0.9177
1.4	0.9192	0.9207	0.9222	0.9236	0.9251	0.9265	0.9279	0.9292	0.9306	0.9319
1.5	0.9332	0.9345	0.9357	0.9370	0.9382	0.9394	0.9406	0.9418	0.9429	0.9441
1.6	0.9452	0.9463	0.9474	0.9484	0.9495	0.9505	0.9515	0.9525	0.9535	0.9545
1.7	0.9554	0.9564	0.9573	0.9582	0.9591	0.9599	0.9608	0.9616	0.9625	0.9633
1.8	0.9641	0.9649	0.9656	0.9664	0.9671	0.9678	0.9686	0.9693	0.9699	0.9706
1.9	0.9713	0.9719	0.9726	0.9732	0.9738	0.9744	0.9750	0.9756	0.9761	0.9767
2.0	0.9772	0.9778	0.9783	0.9788	0.9793	0.9798	0.9803	0.9808	0.9812	0.9817
2.1	0.9821	0.9826	0.9830	0.9834	0.9838	0.9842	0.9846	0.9850	0.9854	0.9857
2.2	0.9861	0.9864	0.9868	0.9871	0.9875	0.9878	0.9881	0.9884	0.9887	0.9890
2.3	0.9893	0.9896	0.9898	0.9901	0.9904	0.9906	0.9909	0.9911	0.9913	0.9916
2.4	0.9918	0.9920	0.9922	0.9925	0.9927	0.9929	0.9931	0.9932	0.9934	0.9936
2.5	0.9938	0.9940	0.9941	0.9943	0.9945	0.9946	0.9948	0.9949	0.9951	0.9952
2.6	0.9953	0.9955	0.9956	0.9957	0.9959	0.9960	0.9961	0.9962	0.9963	0.9964
2.7	0.9965	0.9966	0.9967	0.9968	0.9969	0.9970	0.9971	0.9972	0.9973	0.9974
2.8	0.9974	0.9975	0.9976	0.9977	0.9977	0.9978	0.9979	0.9979	0.9980	0.9981
2.9	0.9981	0.9982	0.9982	0.9983	0.9984	0.9984	0.9985	0.9985	0.9986	0.9986
3.0	0.9987	0.9987	0.9987	0.9988	0.9988	0.9989	0.9989	0.9989	0.9990	0.9990
3.1	0.9990	0.9991	0.9991	0.9991	0.9992	0.9992	0.9992	0.9992	0.9993	0.9993
3.2	0.9993	0.9993	0.9994	0.9994	0.9994	0.9994	0.9994	0.9995	0.9995	0.9995
3.3	0.9995	0.9995	0.9995	0.9996	0.9996	0.9996	0.9996	0.9996	0.9996	0.9997
3.4	0.9997	0.9997	0.9997	0.9997	0.9997	0.9997	0.9997	0.9997	0.9997	0.9998

Adapted from: Pearson, E.S.; Hartley, H.O.: Biometrika tables for statisticians, vol. 1, pp. 110–116 (Biometrika Trustees, Cambridge University Press, London 1954). It appears here with the kind permission of the publishers.

8.5. Using Normal Tables

We have already discovered, in §8.2, that probabilities for $X \sim N(\mu, \sigma^2)$ can be evaluated by computing the equivalent probabilities for the standardized random variable $Z = \frac{X-\mu}{\sigma} \sim N(0, 1)$. Therefore, to calculate any probability for a normal distribution, we only require a table of values of the cumulative probability curve for $Z \sim N(0, 1)$. Such a table of values would still be fairly large if we neglect to exploit additional properties of the standardized normal distribution. Since the total amount of probability in the distribution of Z is always one, it follows that if z is any number we choose, $Pr(Z > z) = 1 - Pr(Z \leqslant z)$; therefore, if a table for the standardized normal distribution specifies the values of $Pr(Z \leqslant z)$ as z varies, we can always calculate $Pr(Z > z)$. More important, since the standardized normal distribution is symmetric about zero, we only need a table of values for $Pr(Z \leqslant z)$ when $z \geqslant 0$ because

$Pr(Z < -z) = Pr(Z > z) = 1 - Pr(Z \leqslant z).$

Table 8.2 specifies values of the cumulative probability curve, $Pr(Z \leqslant z) = \Phi(z)$, for the standardized normal random variable Z. Here we have introduced the symbol $\Phi(z)$ to represent the value of the cumulative probability curve at z. The entry in the table at the intersection of the row labelled 2.5 and the column labelled 0.02 is the value of $\Phi(2.50 + 0.02) = \Phi(2.52) = Pr(Z \leqslant 2.52) = 0.9941$. To calculate the probability that Z is at most 1.56, say, locate $Pr(Z \leqslant 1.56) = \Phi(1.56)$ at the intersection of the row labelled 1.5 and the column labelled 0.06, since $1.56 = 1.50 + 0.06$; the value of $\Phi(1.56)$ is 0.9406. Similarly, $\Phi(0.74) = 0.7704$ and $\Phi(2.32) = 0.9898$. To evaluate $\Phi(-0.74)$ and $\Phi(-2.32)$, we must use the fact that if $z \geqslant 0$,

$\Phi(-z) = Pr(Z \leqslant -z) = Pr(Z \geqslant z) = 1 - Pr(Z < z) = 1 - \Phi(z).$

Then, $\Phi(-0.74) = 1 - \Phi(0.74) = 1 - 0.7704 = 0.2296$ and $\Phi(-2.32) = 1 - \Phi(2.32) = 1 - 0.9898 = 0.0102$.

To calculate $Pr(a < Z < b)$, where a and b are two numbers, we proceed as follows:

$Pr(a < Z < b) = Pr(Z < b) - Pr(Z \leqslant a) = \Phi(b) - \Phi(a).$

Thus, if $a = 1.0$ and $b = 2.5$ we have

$Pr(1.0 < Z < 2.5) = \Phi(2.5) - \Phi(1.0) = 0.9938 - 0.8413 = 0.1525.$

Similarly, when $a = -1.0$ and $b = 2.5$ we obtain

$Pr(-1.0 < Z < 2.5) = \Phi(2.5) - \Phi(-1.0)$
$$= 0.9938 - (1 - \Phi(1.0)) = 0.9938 - 0.1587 = 0.8351.$$

Thus far, we have only used Table 8.2 to calculate probabilities for $Z \sim N(0, 1)$. To handle probabilities for $X \sim N(\mu, \sigma^2)$, we need to use the standardizing transformation, i.e., $\frac{X-\mu}{\sigma} = Z \sim N(0, 1)$. Provided we know the values of μ and σ, we can write

$$\Pr(X \leqslant x) = \Pr\left(\frac{X-\mu}{\sigma} \leqslant \frac{x-\mu}{\sigma}\right) = \Pr\left(Z \leqslant \frac{x-\mu}{\sigma}\right) = \Phi\left(\frac{x-\mu}{\sigma}\right).$$

For example, if $X \sim N(4, 25)$, i.e., $\mu = 4$, $\sigma = 5$, then

$$\Pr(X \leqslant 4) = \Pr\left(Z \leqslant \frac{4-4}{5}\right) = \Phi(0) = 0.500.$$

Likewise,

$$\Pr(X \leqslant 2) = \Pr\left(Z \leqslant \frac{2-4}{5}\right) = \Phi(-0.40) = 1 - \Phi(0.40) = 0.3446.$$

As a final example in the use of normal tables, we evaluate $\Pr(X > 8.49)$ when $X \sim N(3.21, 3.58)$, i.e., $\mu = 3.21$, $\sigma = \sqrt{3.58} = 1.892$:

$$\Pr(X > 8.49) = \Pr\left(Z > \frac{8.49 - 3.21}{1.892}\right) = \Pr(Z > 2.79) = 1 - \Phi(2.79) = 0.0026.$$

9 Analyzing Normally Distributed Data

9.1. Introduction

The methods described in this chapter feature prominently in most introductory textbooks on statistics. In areas of research such as the physical sciences and engineering, measurements are frequently made on a continuous scale. The assumption that such data have a normal distribution has often proved to be a satisfactory description of the observed variation. Methodology for analyzing normally distributed data is therefore important, and deserves its widespread use.

The nature of the data collected in clinical research often precludes the use of these specialized techniques. Consequently, we have emphasized simple methods of analysis which are appropriate for the type of data frequently seen in medical research, especially that concerned with chronic disease. While it is true that none of the material in this chapter is critical to an understanding of the rest of the book, statistical techniques for normally distributed data can be quite useful, and we would be negligent if we failed to mention them altogether. Nonetheless, the discussion involves more formulae than we usually include in one chapter, and readers who find it too taxing should proceed to chapter 10.

Table 9.1 presents the results of an immunological assay carried out on 14 hemophiliacs and 33 normal controls; the test was performed at two concentrations, low and high. The primary purpose of the study was to ascertain if immunological differences between hemophiliacs and normal individuals could be detected. This is one type of data arising in medical research for which the use of statistical techniques for data from a normal distribution may be appropriate. Throughout this chapter, these data will be used to illustrate the methods of analysis which will be discussed.

Table 9.1. The results of an immunological assay of 33 normal controls and 14 hemophiliacs

Controls				Hemophiliacs	
concentration		concentration		concentration	
low	high	low	high	low	high
13.5	25.2	49.2	60.7	11.0	29.0
16.9	44.8	71.5	76.1	9.8	20.3
38.3	62.3	23.3	31.5	61.2	71.2
23.2	47.1	46.1	74.7	63.4	89.9
27.6	39.8	44.5	70.6	11.1	32.4
22.1	44.6	49.4	63.6	8.0	9.9
33.4	54.1	27.2	35.2	40.9	64.3
55.0	55.5	30.6	49.8	47.7	79.1
66.9	86.2	26.1	41.3	19.3	40.2
78.6	102.1	71.5	129.3	18.0	33.7
36.3	88.2	26.6	66.6	24.6	51.8
66.6	68.0	36.9	32.4	39.6	61.4
53.0	92.5	49.5	59.4	24.4	39.3
49.7	73.6	32.8	58.9	11.3	32.8
26.7	40.3	7.9	32.4		
62.9	93.8	9.6	30.0		
46.4	65.4				

9.2. Some Preliminary Considerations

9.2.1. Checking the Normal Assumption

A number of statisticians have investigated the robustness of methods for analyzing normal data. In general, the results of this research suggest that even if the distribution of the data is moderately non-normal, the use of specialized methods for normally distributed data is unlikely to seriously misrepresent the true situation. Nevertheless, it is patently careless to apply the techniques of §9.3–9.5 to a set of observations without first checking that the assumption of a normal distribution for those observations is reasonable, or at least roughly true. Despite the appropriateness of these specialized methods in diverse circumstances, it is probably also true that the same techniques are frequently used in biological settings where the assumption of a normal distribution is not justified.

There are a number of ways in which the reasonableness of the normal distribution assumption may be verified. Perhaps the most straightforward approach involves comparing a histogram for the data with the shape of the normal probability curve. In §1.2, we briefly described how to construct a histogram for a set of data. More detailed instructions can always be found in any elementary text on statistics. Despite the degree of subjectivity which is involved in constructing a histogram, e.g., in the choice of intervals, etc., it is wise to conclude that if the histogram does not appear roughly normal, then the use of methods which are described in this chapter may not be appropriate.

Figure 9.1a presents histograms of the high and low concentration assay results for the control samples, cf. Table 9.1. We can see that the shapes of these two histograms are not radically different from the characteristic shape of a normal probability curve. However, a few large assay values give the histograms a certain asymmetry which is not characteristic of the normal distribution. To correct this problem, one might consider transforming the data. For example, Figure 9.1b shows histograms for the logarithms of the high and low concentration assay results. On a log scale, the large values are perhaps less extreme, but the shapes of the corresponding histograms are not much closer to the characteristic shape of the normal distribution than those of the original data. Although other transformations could be tried, the histograms in Figure 9.1a are not sufficiently non-normal to preclude at least a tentative assumption that the data are normally distributed. Therefore, we will proceed from this assumption and regard the measured values as normal observations. In §9.4.1, the need to use a transformation will be more apparent.

9.2.2. Estimating the Mean and Variance

Except in unusual circumstances where relevant prior information is available concerning the population, the mean, μ, and the variance, σ^2, will need to be estimated from the data. A natural estimate of the population mean is the sample mean. Symbolically, if x_i represents the ith observation in a sample of n values, so that $x_1, x_2, \ldots, x_n$ represent the entire sample, then the formula for $\hat{\mu}$, the estimator of the population mean μ, is

$$\hat{\mu} = \bar{x} = \frac{1}{n} \sum_{i=1}^{n} x_i = \frac{1}{n} (x_1 + x_2 + \ldots + x_n).$$

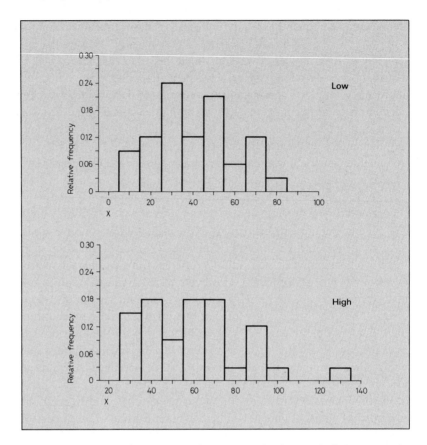

Fig. 9.1a. Histograms of the low and high concentration immunological assay results for the control sample of 33 individuals. Original data.

In §1.3, we described the variance of a distribution as the expected value of the constructed random variable $\{X - E(X)\}^2 = (X - \mu)^2$. If we knew the value of μ, the mean of the distribution, a natural estimate of the population variance, σ^2, would be

$$\frac{1}{n} \sum_{i=1}^{n} (x_i - \mu)^2 = \frac{1}{n} \{(x_1 - \mu)^2 + (x_2 - \mu)^2 + \ldots + (x_n - \mu)^2\}.$$

Since we do not know the value of μ, we can substitute $\hat{\mu} = \bar{x}$ in the above formula. We should realize that this substitution introduces additional uncertainty into our estimate of σ^2, since $\hat{\mu}$ is only an estimate of μ. For reasons

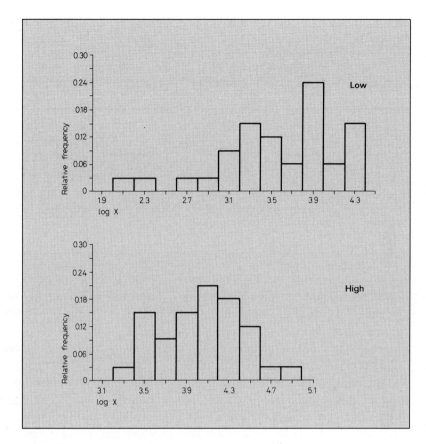

Fig. 9.1b. Logarithms of the original data.

which we cannot explain here, the use of $\bar{x}$ also leads to the replacement of n by (n – 1) in the divisor. The formula for s^2, the estimator of the population variance, σ^2, then becomes

$$s^2 = \frac{1}{n-1} \sum_{i=1}^{n} (x_i - \bar{x})^2 = \frac{1}{n-1} \{(x_1 - \bar{x})^2 + (x_2 - \bar{x})^2 + \ldots + (x_n - \bar{x})^2\}.$$

After a certain amount of algebraic manipulation, this formula can be rewritten as

$$s^2 = \frac{1}{n-1} \left\{ \left(\sum_{i=1}^{n} x_i^2 \right) - n\bar{x}^2 \right\}.$$

Table 9.2. Sample means and sample standard errors for the immunological assay results presented in Table 9.1

	Low concentration		High concentration	
	controls	hemophiliacs	controls	hemophiliacs
n	33	14	33	14
$\Sigma\, x_i$	1319.8	390.3	1996.0	655.3
$\Sigma\, x_i^2$	64212.98	15710.21	138906.30	37768.87
$\bar{x}$	39.99	27.88	60.48	46.81
s^2	357.16	371.48	568.08	545.86
s	18.90	19.27	23.83	23.36

Example calculation: controls, low concentration

$\bar{x} = \frac{1319.8}{33} = 39.99$, $s^2 = \frac{1}{32}\{64212.98 - 33(39.99)^2\} = 357.16$, $s = \sqrt{357.16} = 18.90$.

Both formulae are correct; however, the second expression simplifies the amount of calculation considerably. To estimate the standard error of the data we simply use s, the positive square root of s^2.

From the statistical point of view, $\bar{x}$ and s^2 are, in some sense, the best estimates of μ and σ^2 which we can obtain from the data, i.e., from $x_1, x_2, \ldots, x_n$. These estimates are frequently used for many different types of data; however, it is wise to remember that they are not necessarily good estimates of the mean and variance for every possible probability distribution.

Table 9.2 shows the detailed calculations which lead to the estimates $\bar{x}$ and s for the low and high concentration assay results presented in Table 9.1. The values of $\bar{x}$ and s could be used to estimate a plausible range of values for the immunological test procedure; however, this information does not explicitly address the question of immunological differences between the hemophiliac and control populations. To investigate this question, we require the methods which are described in §9.4.

9.3. Analyzing a Single Sample

In most practical circumstances involving a single sample from a particular population, the principal question which is of interest concerns the value of μ, the population mean. Either we may wish to test the hypothesis that μ is equal to a specific value μ_0, say, or we may wish to derive a confidence interval for μ. We know that the sample average is a natural estimate of μ. Therefore, it should not be surprising that the sample average is used to test the hypothesis H: $\mu = \mu_0$, and also to derive a suitable confidence interval for μ.

If we let the random variables X_1, X_2, ..., X_n represent a single sample of n observations, then the assumption that these data are normally distributed can be specified, symbolically, by writing $X_i \sim N(\mu, \sigma^2)$ for $i = 1, 2, ...,$ n. It can also be shown that the sample average, $\overline{X} = \frac{1}{n} \sum_{i=1}^{n} X_i$, has a normal distribution with mean μ and variance σ^2/n, i.e., $\overline{X} \sim N(\mu, \sigma^2/n)$. Therefore, the standardizing transformation of chapter 8 guarantees that

$$Z = \frac{\overline{X} - \mu}{\sigma/\sqrt{n}} \sim N(0, 1),$$

and a suitable test statistic for evaluating the significance level of the data with respect to the hypothesis H: $\mu = \mu_0$ is

$$T = \frac{|\overline{X} - \mu_0|}{\sigma/\sqrt{n}}.$$

If σ is known and t_0 is the observed value of T, then the significance level of the test is $Pr(T \geq t_0)$. As we discovered in §8.4, the calculations which generate a confidence interval for μ are based on the fact that $T = |Z|$, where $Z \sim N(0, 1)$. The formula specifying a 95% confidence interval for μ is the interval

$$(\overline{x} - 1.96\,\sigma/\sqrt{n}, \overline{x} + 1.96\,\sigma/\sqrt{n}),$$

where $\overline{x}$ is the observed sample mean.

In most cases, σ will not be known. An obvious solution to this problem involves replacing σ by its estimate, s. In this case, the significance level is only approximate, since $Z = \frac{\overline{X} - \mu_0}{s/\sqrt{n}}$ no longer has a normal distribution; we have estimated σ by s. However, if the number of observations is large, i.e., $n \geq 50$, the approximation will be quite accurate. Similar comments apply to the approximate 95% confidence interval $(\overline{x} - 1.96\,s/\sqrt{n}, \overline{x} + 1.96\,s/\sqrt{n})$.

If we apply these methods to the immunological data discussed in §9.1, 9.2, we obtain two approximate 95% confidence intervals for the mean assay results in each of the study groups. The results of these calculations are given in Table 9.3. Since there is no previous information regarding these assays in either the hemophiliacs or the controls, there is no natural hypothesis concerning μ, i.e., no obvious value μ_0, that we might consider testing with these data.

In the preceding discussion, we remarked that when σ is replaced by s in the formula for T and the corresponding 95% confidence interval for μ, the

Table 9.3. Approximate 95% confidence intervals for the mean immunological assay results, at low and high concentrations, in the hemophiliac and control populations

	Concentration	
	low	high
Controls	(33.54, 46.44)	(52.35, 68.61)
Hemophiliacs	(17.79, 37.97)	(34.57, 59.05)

Example calculation: controls, low concentration (n = 33)

$\bar{x} = 39.99$ $1.96s/\sqrt{n} = \frac{1.96(18.90)}{\sqrt{33}} = 6.45$

$s = 18.90$ $\bar{x} - 6.45 = 33.54, \ \bar{x} + 6.45 = 46.44$.

results we obtain are only approximate. This is because s is an estimate of σ. As a result, we are more uncertain about the precise value of μ. In particular, if the sample size is rather small, e.g., n < 30, say, we ought to use the exact distribution of $T = \frac{|\bar{X} - \mu_0|}{s/\sqrt{n}}$ to calculate the significance level of the data with respect to the hypothesis H: $\mu = \mu_0$, and also to obtain a 95% confidence interval for μ. Now if the null hypothesis is true, it can be shown that the statistic $\frac{\bar{X} - \mu_0}{s/\sqrt{n}}$ has a Student's t distribution on (n−1) degrees of freedom; symbolically, we write this as $\frac{\bar{X} - \mu_0}{s/\sqrt{n}} \sim t_{(n-1)}$. The probability curve for the Student's t distribution is similar to that of the standardized normal distribution. Both curves are symmetric about zero and are approximately bell-shaped; however, the curve for $t_{(n-1)}$ is somewhat more spread out than the probability curve of Z. In fact, the spread of the Student's t distribution depends on a parameter called the degrees of freedom. Since this parameter is equal to (n−1), i.e., sample size minus one, the degrees of freedom reflect the number of observations used to estimate σ and, therefore, how accurate an estimate s is likely to be. A Student's t distribution with large degrees of freedom, say 50, is virtually indistinguishable from a standardized normal distribution.

   Statistical tables for the Student's t distribution are usually drawn up on the same principle as a table of critical values for the distribution of $|Z|$ (cf., Table 8.1). Each row of the table corresponds to an integer value of the degrees of freedom, and each column of the table represents a specified probability level; thus, the values in the body of the table are critical values for the distribution of $T = |t_{(k)}|$. For an example of Student's t distribution tables which correspond to this format, see Table 9.4. Critical values for the distri-

Table 9.4. Critical values of the probability distribution of $T = |t_{(k)}|$; the table specifies values of the number t_o such that $Pr(T \geqslant t_o) = p$

Degrees of freedom (k)	Probability level, p					
	0.10	0.05	0.02	0.01	0.002	0.001
1	6.314	12.706	31.82	63.66	318.3	636.6
2	2.920	4.303	6.695	9.925	22.33	31.60
3	2.353	3.182	4.541	5.841	10.21	12.92
4	2.132	2.776	3.747	4.604	7.173	8.610
5	2.015	2.571	3.365	4.032	5.893	6.869
6	1.943	2.447	3.143	3.707	5.208	5.959
7	1.895	2.365	2.998	3.499	4.785	5.408
8	1.860	2.306	2.896	3.355	4.501	5.041
9	1.833	2.262	2.821	3.250	4.297	4.781
10	1.812	2.228	2.764	3.169	4.144	4.587
11	1.796	2.201	2.718	3.106	4.025	4.437
12	1.782	2.179	2.681	3.055	3.930	4.318
13	1.771	2.160	2.650	3.012	3.852	4.221
14	1.761	2.145	2.624	2.977	3.787	4.140
15	1.753	2.131	2.602	2.947	3.733	4.073
16	1.746	2.120	2.583	2.921	3.686	4.015
17	1.740	2.110	2.567	2.898	3.646	3.965
18	1.734	2.101	2.552	2.878	3.610	3.922
19	1.729	2.093	2.539	2.861	3.579	3.883
20	1.725	2.086	2.528	2.845	3.552	3.850
21	1.721	2.080	2.518	2.831	3.527	3.819
22	1.717	2.074	2.508	2.819	3.505	3.792
23	1.714	2.069	2.500	2.807	3.485	3.767
24	1.711	2.064	2.492	2.797	3.467	3.745
25	1.708	2.060	2.485	2.787	3.450	3.725
26	1.706	2.056	2.479	2.779	3.435	3.707
27	1.703	2.052	2.473	2.771	3.421	3.690
28	1.701	2.048	2.467	2.763	3.408	3.674
29	1.699	2.045	2.462	2.756	3.396	3.659
30	1.697	2.042	2.457	2.750	3.385	3.646
40	1.684	2.021	2.423	2.704	3.307	3.551
60	1.671	2.000	2.390	2.660	3.232	3.460
120	1.658	1.980	2.358	2.617	3.160	3.373
∞ (normal)	1.645	1.960	2.326	2.576	3.090	3.291

Abridged from Pearson, E.S.; Hartley, H.O.: Biometrika tables for statisticians, vol. 1, p. 146 (Biometrika Trustees, Cambridge University Press, London 1954). It appears here with the kind permission of the publishers.

bution of $|Z|$ may be found in the last row of Table 9.4, since a $t_{(\infty)}$ distribution is identical with the distribution of Z. Notice that these values are all smaller than the corresponding critical values found in other rows of the table; this difference reflects the fact that the Student's t distribution is more variable than the standardized normal distribution.

A suitable test statistic for evaluating the significance level of the data with respect to the hypothesis H: $\mu = \mu_0$ is

$$T = \frac{|\overline{X} - \mu_0|}{s/\sqrt{n}};$$

since $\frac{\overline{X} - \mu_0}{s/\sqrt{n}} \sim t_{(n-1)}$ if the null hypothesis is true, it follows that $T \sim |t_{(n-1)}|$. Therefore, if t_o is the observed value of T, the significance level is equal to

$$Pr(T \geq t_o) = Pr(|t_{(n-1)}| \geq t_o);$$

this is the reason that Table 9.4 presents critical values of the distribution of $T = |t_{(k)}|$. Similar calculations lead to the formula

$$(\overline{x} - t^* s/\sqrt{n}, \overline{x} + t^* s/\sqrt{n}),$$

which specifies a 95% confidence interval for μ, where t^* is the appropriate 5% critical value from Table 9.4, i.e., $Pr(T \geq t^*) = Pr(|t_{(n-1)}| \geq t^*) = 0.05$. Notice that this version of the 95% confidence interval for μ differs from the approximate confidence interval which we obtained at the beginning of this section only in the replacement of 1.96, the 5% critical value for $|Z|$, by t^*, the corresponding critical value for the distribution of $T = |t_{(n-1)}|$. Replacing 1.96 by t^* always increases the width of the confidence interval, since t^* exceeds 1.96. The increased width reflects our increased uncertainty concerning plausible values of μ since we have used s, an estimate of σ, to derive the 95% confidence interval.

Exact 95% confidence intervals for the mean assay results at low and high concentrations in the hemophiliac and control populations may be found in Table 9.5; the table also shows selected details of the calculations. If we compare corresponding intervals in Tables 9.3 and 9.5, we see that the exact 95% confidence interval is always wider than the corresponding approximate confidence interval. Since the separate 95% confidence intervals for hemophiliacs and controls overlap at both the low and high concentrations, we might reasonably conclude that, at each concentration level, the data do not contradict the hypothesis that the mean assay in the two populations is the same. An alternative method for investigating this question, which is essentially the problem of comparing two means in normally distributed data, is discussed in §9.4.

Table 9.5. Exact 95% confidence intervals for the mean immunological assay results, at low and high concentrations, in the hemophiliac and control populations

	Concentration	
	low	high
Controls	(33.27, 46.71)	(52.01, 68.95)
Hemophiliacs	(16.76, 39.00)	(33.32, 60.30)

| Example calculations: | low concentration |

Hemophiliacs (n = 14):

$\bar{x} = 27.88$

$s = 19.27$

$$2.160s/\sqrt{n} = \frac{2.160(19.27)}{\sqrt{14}} = 11.12^a$$

$$\bar{x} - 11.12 = 16.76, \quad \bar{x} + 11.12 = 39.00$$

Controls (n = 33):

$\bar{x} = 39.99$

$s = 18.90$

$$2.042s/\sqrt{n} = \frac{2.042(18.90)}{\sqrt{33}} = 6.72^b$$

$$\bar{x} - 6.72 = 33.27, \quad \bar{x} + 6.72 = 46.71$$

[a] The 5% critical value for $|t_{(13)}|$ is 2.160 (see Table 9.4).
[b] Since the 5% critical value for $|t_{(32)}|$ is not given in Table 9.4, we use the corresponding value for $|t_{(30)}|$, which is 2.042.

9.4. Comparisons Based on the Normal Distribution

9.4.1. Paired Data

In previous chapters, we discussed the importance of stratifying data in order to properly evaluate comparisons that were of interest. The basic premise of stratification is that any comparison with respect to a particular factor should be made between groups which are alike with respect to other factors that may influence the response. Data which are naturally paired constitute a special case of stratification, and typically facilitate a more precise comparison than might otherwise be achieved. Before and after measurements are perhaps the most common illustration of naturally paired data; for example, we might wish to investigate the efficacy of an anti-hypertensive drug by using measurements of a patient's blood pressure before and after the drug is administered. In another circumstance, if we had identical twins who differed with respect to smoking status, we might consider measuring several aspects of lung function in each twin in order to investigate the effect of smoking on lung function.

When data involve natural pairing, a common method of analysis is based on the assumption that the differences between the paired observations are normally distributed. If we let the random variables $D_1, D_2, ..., D_n$ represent these differences, e.g., Before-After, then we are assuming that $D_i \sim N(\mu_d, \sigma_d^2)$ for i = 1, 2, ..., n; μ_d is the mean difference in response, and σ_d^2 is the variance of the differences. Provided this assumption is reasonable, then all the methods for a single sample of normally distributed data can be used to analyze the differences. For example, a natural hypothesis to test in this situation would be H: $\mu_d = 0$; i.e., the mean difference in response is zero. If the data provide evidence to contradict this hypothesis, then we would conclude that the factor which varies within each pair, e.g., smoking status, or use of the anti-hypertensive drug, has a real effect. We might also want to evaluate a suitable confidence interval for μ_d in order to estimate the magnitude and direction of the effect which has been detected.

The immunological data which we have previously discussed do involve natural pairing since, for each subject, we have one assay result at each concentration level. If we compute the High-Low differences of the assay results for each patient, we could separately investigate the effect of concentration among hemophiliacs, and also among the controls. Although this question is not of primary interest to the study, we shall treat the data for the controls as we have described in order to illustrate the analysis of paired observations.

The original assay results may be found in Table 9.1. The difference, High – Low, was calculated for each control subject, yielding 33 observations. A histogram of this sample of differences is given in Figure 9.2a. The distribution of the differences is quite spread out, and one might be reluctant to assume that the distribution is normal. An alternative approach would be to consider the differences in the logarithms of the assay results. This is equivalent to considering the logarithm of the ratio of the assay results. A histogram of the logarithm differences is given in Figure 9.2b, and it can be seen that the shape of this histogram is considerably closer to the characteristic shape of a normal probability curve than that of the histogram in Figure 9.2a. Therefore, we will analyze the differences between the logarithms of the assay results at the two concentrations, and assume that these differences are normally distributed.

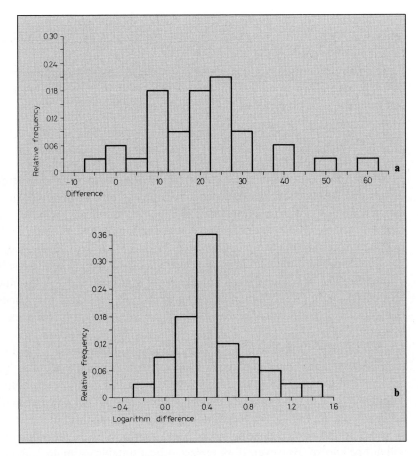

Fig. 9.2. Histograms of the difference in immunological assay results at high and low concentrations for the control sample of 33 individuals. **a** Original data. **b** Logarithms of the original data.

For these logarithm differences we obtain $\bar{x} = 0.47$ and $s = 0.33$. The observed value of T, the statistic for testing H: $\mu_d = 0$, is

$$t_o = \frac{|\bar{x} - 0|}{s/\sqrt{n}} = \frac{0.47}{0.33/\sqrt{33}} = 8.18.$$

As we might expect, this large observed value tells us that the data provide strong evidence to contradict the hypothesis that the mean logarithm difference is zero ($p < 0.001$); we therefore conclude that concentration influences the assay result.

The magnitude of this effect, i.e., the change with concentration, is indicated by the estimated mean of 0.47, and also by the 95% confidence interval for μ_d, which is (0.35, 0.59).

In many circumstances, it is not possible to make comparisons which are based on naturally paired data. Methods which are appropriate for this more common situation are discussed in the next section.

9.4.2. Unpaired Data

If the data are not naturally paired, then the comparison of interest usually involves two separate, independent samples from two (assumed) normal distributions. We can portray this situation, symbolically, by using the random variables $X_1, X_2, \ldots, X_n$ to represent one sample and $Y_1, Y_2, \ldots, Y_m$ to represent the second sample; then $X_i \sim N(\mu_x, \sigma^2)$ for $i = 1, 2, \ldots, n$ and $Y_j \sim N(\mu_y, \sigma^2)$ for $j = 1, 2, \ldots, m$. For example, the X's may be the results of lung function tests for a random sample of smokers, and the Y's may be a corresponding set of observations on nonsmokers. The primary question of interest in such a situation is usually a comparison of the means, μ_x and μ_y.

Since $\overline{X} = \frac{1}{n} \sum_{i=1}^{n} X_i$ and $\overline{Y} = \frac{1}{m} \sum_{j=1}^{m} Y_j$ are natural estimates of μ_x and μ_y, the obvious quantity on which to base a comparison of μ_x and μ_y is $\overline{X} - \overline{Y}$, the difference in sample means. Conveniently, $\overline{X} - \overline{Y}$ has a normal distribution with mean $(\mu_x - \mu_y)$ and variance $\sigma^2(1/n + 1/m)$. When σ is known, a confidence interval for $(\mu_x - \mu_y)$ or a significance test concerning this difference can be based on the normal distribution of $\overline{X} - \overline{Y}$. In most cases, the value of σ will not be known. However, if we replace σ by a suitable estimate, s, then it can be shown that

$$\frac{\overline{X} - \overline{Y} - (\mu_x - \mu_y)}{s\sqrt{1/n + 1/m}} \sim t_{(n + m - 2)}.$$

In view of the results which we described in §9.3, this is the distribution that we would expect to obtain after replacing σ by s. To estimate σ^2, the common variance in the two populations, we use a weighted average of

$$s_x^2 = \frac{1}{n-1} \sum_{i=1}^{n} (x_i - \overline{x})^2 = \frac{1}{n-1} \left\{ \sum_{i=1}^{n} x_i^2 - n\overline{x}^2 \right\}$$

and

$$s_y^2 = \frac{1}{m-1} \sum_{j=1}^{m} (y_j - \overline{y})^2 = \frac{1}{m-1} \left\{ \sum_{j=1}^{m} y_j^2 - m\overline{y}^2 \right\},$$

the individual sample estimates. The formula for the combined or pooled estimate of σ^2 is

$$s^2 = \frac{(n-1)s_x^2 + (m-1)s_y^2}{n + m - 2}.$$

To test the hypothesis that $(\mu_x - \mu_y)$ is equal to μ_0, say, we would use the test statistic

$$T = \frac{|\overline{X} - \overline{Y} - \mu_0|}{s\sqrt{1/n + 1/m}}.$$

In many circumstances it is the hypothesis of equal means, H: $\mu_x = \mu_y$, i.e., $\mu_x - \mu_y = \mu_0 = 0$, which is of primary interest. If the null hypothesis is true, $T \sim |t_{(n+m-2)}|$. Therefore, if t_0 is the observed value of T, the significance level of the data is equal to $\Pr(T \geq t_0) = \Pr(|t_{(n+m-2)}| \geq t_0)$; this value can be estimated using Table 9.4.

If a 95% confidence interval for $(\mu_x - \mu_y)$ is required, the formula which is obtained from the usual calculations is

$$(\overline{x} - \overline{y} - t^*s\sqrt{1/n + 1/m} \,, \overline{x} - \overline{y} + t^*s\sqrt{1/n + 1/m}),$$

where $\overline{x}$ and $\overline{y}$ are the observed sample means, and t^* is the appropriate 5% critical value from Table 9.4, i.e., $\Pr(T \geq t^*) = \Pr(|t_{(n+m-2)}| \geq t^*) = 0.05$.

The purpose of the immunological study was to characterize differences between the hemophiliacs and the controls. The techniques for unpaired data which we have just described allow us to address this question explicitly. We shall look, separately, at the two concentration levels, using X's to represent the assay results for hemophiliacs and Y's for the results in the controls; summary statistics for each group may be found in Table 9.6. A natural hypothesis to test in this data set is H: $\mu_x = \mu_y$, i.e., $\mu_x - \mu_y = 0$. Details of the actual calculations which are required to test this hypothesis, at each concentration, may be found in Table 9.6.

The significance level for a test of the hypothesis that $\mu_x = \mu_y$ is $\Pr(|t_{(45)}| \geq t_0)$, where t_0 is the observed value of the test statistic. Since there is no row in Table 9.4 corresponding to 45 degrees of freedom, we compare t_0 with the 5% critical values for both 40 and 60 degrees of freedom. These values are 2.021 and 2.00, respectively. For the low concentration results, the value of t_0 is 2.00, which corresponds, approximately, to a significance level of 0.05. The observed value of the test statistic for the high concentration assays is 1.81, which lies between the 5 and 10% critical values for both 40 and 60 degrees of freedom; thus, the p-value associated with this test of significance is between 0.05 and 0.10. From these results we conclude that

Table 9.6. Comparing the mean immunological assay results, at low and high concentrations, in the hemophiliac and control populations

	Concentration	
	low	high
Hemophiliacs (n = 14)	$\bar{x} = 27.88$, $s_x^2 = 371.48$	$\bar{x} = 46.81$, $s_x^2 = 545.86$
Controls (m = 33)	$\bar{y} = 39.99$, $s_y^2 = 357.16$	$\bar{y} = 60.48$, $s_y^2 = 568.08$
Pooled estimate, $s^2 = \dfrac{13s_x^2 + 32s_y^2}{45}$	$\dfrac{13(371.48) + 32(357.16)}{45} = 361.30$	$\dfrac{13(545.86) + 32(568.08)}{45} = 561.66$
Observed value, $t_o = \dfrac{\lvert\bar{x}-\bar{y}\rvert}{s\sqrt{1/14 + 1/33}}$	$\dfrac{\lvert 27.88 - 39.99\rvert}{19.01\sqrt{1/14 + 1/33}} = 2.00$	$\dfrac{\lvert 46.81 - 60.48\rvert}{23.70\sqrt{1/14 + 1/33}} = 1.81$
Significance level, $\Pr(\lvert t_{(45)}\rvert \geqslant t_o)$	0.05	0.05 – 0.10
95% confidence interval for $(\mu_x - \mu_y)$, $(\bar{x} - \bar{y}) \pm 2.021\, s\sqrt{1/14 + 1/33}$[a]	(−24.36, 0.14)	(−28.95, 1.61)

[a] Since the 5% critical value for $\lvert t_{(45)}\rvert$ is not given in Table 9.4, we use the corresponding value for $\lvert t_{(40)}\rvert$, which is 2.021.

there is suggestive evidence, at both low and high concentrations, for different mean assay results in the two populations. The 95% confidence intervals for $(\mu_x - \mu_y)$ which are given in Table 9.6 include zero near the upper endpoint of each interval, and are consistent with this conclusion concerning μ_x and μ_y.

Notice that the evidence concerning different population mean values is somewhat stronger in Table 9.6 than that which might be derived from an informal comparison of the confidence intervals presented in Table 9.5. This is because the analysis summarized in Table 9.6 uses the pooled estimate of variance, which will be more accurate than the use of two separate variance estimates, as in Table 9.5. A method for examining the validity of the pooled estimate is described in the next section.

9.5. Testing the Equality of Variances

A critical assumption in the analysis of unpaired data which we described in §9.4.2 is the requirement that the variance in each population is the common value σ^2. It is difficult to imagine a situation where this requirement could be assumed to hold without checking its reasonableness. Let us suppose that $X_1, X_2, \ldots, X_n$ and $Y_1, Y_2, \ldots, Y_m$ represent unpaired samples of normally distributed observations. If s_x^2 and s_y^2 are the sample estimates of the variances σ_x^2 and σ_y^2, then the appropriate statistic for testing the hypothesis that the variances are equal, i.e., H: $\sigma_x^2 = \sigma_y^2 = \sigma^2$, is the ratio

$$R = \frac{s_x^2}{s_y^2},$$

where s_x^2 is assumed to be greater than s_y^2. If s_y^2 exceeds s_x^2, then the roles of the two samples can simply be interchanged.

If the null hypothesis that $\sigma_x^2 = \sigma_y^2 = \sigma^2$ is true, the ratio R has a probability distribution which depends on the F-distribution. This latter distribution is characterized by two parameters, the degrees of freedom associated with s_x^2, the greater variance estimate, and the degrees of freedom associated with s_y^2, the lesser variance estimate. Since the values of s_x^2 and s_y^2 were calculated from n and m observations, respectively, the corresponding degrees of freedom are $(n-1)$ and $(m-1)$. Therefore, if the null hypothesis is true, and if r_0 is the observed value of R, the significance level of the data is equal to

$$Pr(R \geqslant r_0) = 2Pr(F_{n-1, m-1} \geqslant r_0).$$

Table 9.7a. Selected 5% critical values of the F-distribution; the table gives values of the number r_o such that $Pr(F_{n.m} \geqslant r_o) = 0.05$

Degrees of freedom for the smaller variance estimate (m)	Degrees of freedom for the greater variance estimate (n)							
	1	2	3	4	5	6	12	∞
1	161.4	199.5	215.7	224.6	230.2	234.0	243.9	254.3
2	18.51	19.00	19.16	19.25	19.30	19.33	19.41	19.50
3	10.13	9.55	9.28	9.12	9.01	8.94	8.74	8.53
4	7.71	6.94	6.59	6.39	6.26	6.16	5.91	5.63
5	6.61	5.79	5.41	5.19	5.05	4.95	4.68	4.36
6	5.99	5.14	4.76	4.53	4.39	4.28	4.00	3.67
7	5.59	4.74	4.35	4.12	3.97	3.87	3.57	3.23
8	5.32	4.46	4.07	3.84	3.69	3.58	3.28	2.93
9	5.12	4.26	3.86	3.63	3.48	3.37	3.07	2.71
10	4.96	4.10	3.71	3.48	3.33	3.22	2.91	2.54
11	4.84	3.98	3.59	3.36	3.20	3.09	2.79	2.40
12	4.75	3.89	3.49	3.26	3.11	3.00	2.69	2.30
13	4.67	3.81	3.41	3.18	3.03	2.92	2.60	2.21
14	4.60	3.74	3.34	3.11	2.96	2.85	2.53	2.13
15	4.54	3.68	3.29	3.06	2.90	2.79	2.48	2.07
16	4.49	3.63	3.24	3.01	2.85	2.74	2.42	2.01
17	4.45	3.59	3.20	2.96	2.81	2.70	2.38	1.96
18	4.41	3.55	3.16	2.93	2.77	2.66	2.34	1.92
19	4.38	3.52	3.13	2.90	2.74	2.63	2.31	1.88
20	4.35	3.49	3.10	2.87	2.71	2.60	2.28	1.84
21	4.32	3.47	3.07	2.84	2.68	2.57	2.25	1.81
22	4.30	3.44	3.05	2.82	2.66	2.55	2.23	1.78
23	4.28	3.42	3.03	2.80	2.64	2.53	2.20	1.76
24	4.26	3.40	3.01	2.78	2.62	2.51	2.18	1.73
25	4.24	3.39	2.99	2.76	2.60	2.49	2.16	1.71
26	4.23	3.37	2.98	2.74	2.59	2.47	2.15	1.69
27	4.21	3.35	2.96	2.73	2.57	2.46	2.13	1.67
28	4.20	3.34	2.95	2.71	2.56	2.45	2.12	1.65
29	4.18	3.33	2.93	2.70	2.55	2.43	2.10	1.64
30	4.17	3.32	2.92	2.69	2.53	2.42	2.09	1.62
40	4.08	3.23	2.84	2.61	2.45	2.34	2.00	1.51
60	4.00	3.15	2.76	2.53	2.37	2.25	1.92	1.39
120	3.92	3.07	2.68	2.45	2.29	2.17	1.83	1.25
∞	3.84	3.00	2.60	2.37	2.21	2.10	1.75	1.00

Abridged from Pearson, E.S.; Hartley, H.O.: Biometrika tables for statisticians, vol. 1, p. 171 (Biometrika Trustees, Cambridge University Press, London 1954). It appears here with the kind permission of the publishers.

Table 9.7b. Selected 2.5% critical values of the F-distribution; the table gives values of the number r_0 such that $\Pr(F_{n,m} \geq r_0) = 0.025$

Degrees of freedom for the smaller variance estimate (m)	Degrees of freedom for the greater variance estimate (n)							
	1	2	3	4	5	6	12	∞
1	647.8	799.5	864.2	899.6	921.8	937.1	976.7	1,018
2	38.51	39.00	39.17	39.25	39.30	39.33	39.41	39.50
3	17.44	16.04	15.44	15.10	14.88	14.73	14.34	13.90
4	12.22	10.65	9.98	9.60	9.36	9.20	8.75	8.26
5	10.01	8.43	7.76	7.39	7.15	6.98	6.52	6.02
6	8.81	7.26	6.60	6.23	5.99	5.82	5.37	4.85
7	8.07	6.54	5.89	5.52	5.29	5.12	4.67	4.14
8	7.57	6.06	5.42	5.05	4.82	4.65	4.20	3.67
9	7.21	5.71	5.08	4.72	4.48	4.32	3.87	3.33
10	6.94	5.46	4.83	4.47	4.24	4.07	3.62	3.08
11	6.72	5.26	4.63	4.28	4.04	3.88	3.43	2.88
12	6.55	5.10	4.47	4.12	3.89	3.73	3.28	2.72
13	6.41	4.97	4.35	4.00	3.77	3.60	3.15	2.60
14	6.30	4.86	4.24	3.89	3.66	3.50	3.05	2.49
15	6.20	4.77	4.15	3.80	3.58	3.41	2.96	2.40
16	6.12	4.69	4.08	3.73	3.50	3.34	2.89	2.32
17	6.04	4.62	4.01	3.66	3.44	3.28	2.82	2.25
18	5.98	4.56	3.95	3.61	3.38	3.22	2.77	2.19
19	5.92	4.51	3.90	3.56	3.33	3.17	2.72	2.13
20	5.87	4.46	3.86	3.51	3.29	3.13	2.68	2.09
21	5.83	4.42	3.82	3.48	3.25	3.09	2.64	2.04
22	5.79	4.38	3.78	3.44	3.22	3.05	2.60	2.00
23	5.75	4.35	3.75	3.41	3.18	3.02	2.57	1.97
24	5.72	4.32	3.72	3.38	3.15	2.99	2.54	1.94
25	5.69	4.29	3.69	3.35	3.13	2.97	2.51	1.91
26	5.66	4.27	3.67	3.33	3.10	2.94	2.49	1.88
27	5.63	4.24	3.65	3.31	3.08	2.92	2.47	1.85
28	5.61	4.22	3.63	3.29	3.06	2.90	2.45	1.83
29	5.59	4.20	3.61	3.27	3.04	2.88	2.43	1.81
30	5.57	4.18	3.59	3.25	3.03	2.87	2.41	1.79
40	5.42	4.05	3.46	3.13	2.90	2.74	2.29	1.64
60	5.29	3.93	3.34	3.01	2.79	2.63	2.17	1.48
120	5.15	3.80	3.23	2.89	2.67	2.52	2.05	1.31
∞	5.02	3.69	3.12	2.79	2.57	2.41	1.94	1.00

Abridged from Pearson, E.S.; Hartley, H.O.: Biometrika tables for statisticians, vol. 1, p. 172 (Biometrika Trustees, Cambridge University Press, London 1954). It appears here with the kind permission of the publishers.

Table 9.8. Testing the assumption of equal variances for the distribution of immunological assay results, at low and high concentrations, in the hemophiliac and control populations

---

Low concentration

Hemophiliacs:	$n = 14$	$s_x^2 = 371.48$
Controls:	$m = 33$	$s_y^2 = 357.16$

$$r_0 = \frac{s_x^2}{s_y^2} = \frac{371.48}{357.16} = 1.04$$

$$\Pr(R \geqslant r_0) = 2\Pr(F_{13,32} \geqslant 1.04) > 0.10^a$$

High concentration

Controls:	$n = 33$	$s_x^2 = 568.08$	$r_0 = 1.04$
Hemophiliacs:	$m = 14$	$s_y^2 = 545.86$	

$$\Pr(R \geqslant r_0) = 2\Pr(F_{32,13} \geqslant 1.04) > 0.10^b$$

---

[a] The 5% critical values for $F_{12,30}$ and $F_{12,40}$ are 2.09 and 2.00, respectively.
[b] The 5% critical values for $F_{12,13}$ and $F_{\infty,13}$ are 2.60 and 2.21, respectively.

Table 9.7 gives selected critical values for a number of different F-distributions. In using Table 9.7, or any of the more extensive sets of statistical tables for the F-distribution which are available, an observed value of the ratio R should be compared with the entry in the statistical table which has degrees of freedom closest to $(n-1)$ and $(m-1)$, if an exact match is not possible. The use of more extensive tables will usually permit a more precise determination of the significance level. If the observed value of R is at all large, the appropriateness of any method for analyzing normal data which is based on the common variance assumption is questionable.

In the case of the immunological data, the observed values of R for the high and low concentration assay results can be calculated from the information given in Table 9.6. Details of the calculations which are involved in testing the common variance assumption are presented in Table 9.8. The equal variances assumption is not contradicted by the data at either concentration level.

If the data suggest that the variances in two unpaired samples are apparently different, then it is important to ask whether, in light of this information, a comparison of means is appropriate. A substantial difference in the variances may, in fact, be the most important finding concerning the data. Also, when the variances are different, the difference in means no longer adequately summarizes how the two groups differ.

If, after careful consideration, a comparison of means is still thought to be important, then the appropriate procedure is not uniformly agreed upon among statisticians. The reasons for this disagreement are beyond the scope of this book, but approximate methods should be adequate in most situations. Therefore, we suggest the simple approach of calculating a confidence interval for μ_x and a second interval for μ_y. If these intervals overlap, then the hypothesis that μ_x is equal to μ_y would not be contradicted by the data. If the nature of the practical problem makes this ad hoc approach inappropriate or inadequate, then a statistician should be consulted.

In chapter 10, we will also be discussing a method for analyzing normally distributed data. In fact, the techniques which we have described in chapter 9 can be regarded as a special case of the methodology which is presented in chapter 10. We do not intend to elaborate further on this connection, since the purposes of these two chapters are quite different. Chapter 9 constitutes a brief introduction to material which, although important, is not a primary focus of this book. However, in chapter 10 we introduce a class of statistical techniques which will feature prominently in the remaining chapters. We therefore direct our attention, at this point, to the important topic of regression models.

10 Linear Regression Models for Medical Data

10.1. Introduction

Many medical studies investigate the association of a number of different factors with an outcome of interest. In some of the previous chapters, we discussed methods of studying the role of a single factor, perhaps with stratification according to other factors to account for heterogeneity in the study population. When there is simultaneous interest in more than one factor, these techniques have limited application.

Regression models are frequently used in such multi-factor situations. These models take a variety of forms, but their common aim is to study the joint effect of a number of different factors on an outcome variable. The quantitative nature of the outcome variable often determines the particular choice of regression model. One type of model will be discussed in this chapter. The two succeeding chapters will introduce other regression models. In all three chapters, we intend to emphasize the general nature of these models and the types of questions which they are designed to answer. We hope that the usefulness of regression models will become apparent as our discussion of them proceeds.

Before we launch into a description of linear regression models and how they are used in medical statistics, it is probably important to make a few brief comments about the concept of a statistical model. A relationship such as Einstein's famous equation linking energy and mass, $E = mc^2$, is an exact and true description of the nature of things. Statistical models, however, use equations quite differently. The equation for a statistical model is not expected to be exactly true; instead, it represents a useful framework within which the statistician is able to study relationships which are of interest, such as the association between survival and age, aggressiveness of disease and the treatment which a patient receives. There is frequently no particular biological support for statistical models. In general, they should be regarded simply as an attempt to provide an empirical summary of observed data. Finally, no model can be routinely used without checking that it does indeed provide a reasonable description of the available data.

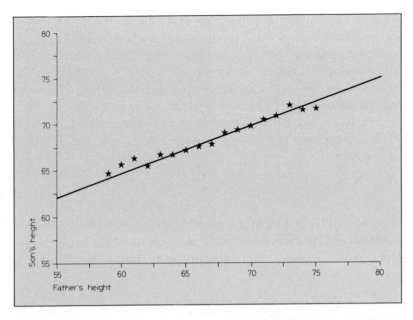

Fig. 10.1. A scatterplot of the data collected by *Pearson and Lee* [1903] concerning the heights of father-son pairs. The equation of the fitted regression line is $\hat{Y} = 33.73 + 0.516X$.

10.2. A Historical Note

The term 'regression' arose in the context of studying the heights of members of family groups. *Pearson and Lee* [1903] collected data on the heights of 1078 father-son pairs in order to study Galton's 'law of universal regression' which states that 'Each peculiarity in a man is shared by his kinsmen, but *on the average* in a less degree'. Figure 10.1 shows a plot of the average height of the sons in each of 17 groups which were defined by first classifying the fathers into 17 groups, using one-inch intervals of height between 58.5 and 75.5 inches.

If we represent the height of a son by the random variable Y, and the height of a father by the random variable X, then the straight line drawn in Figure 10.1 is simply the equation

Son's height = 33.73 + 0.516 × Father's height

or

Y = 33.73 + 0.516 X.   (10.1)

We shall use numbers in parentheses to label equations to which we later wish to refer. Equation (10.1) is called a regression equation. The variable Y is called the dependent or outcome variable, and X is called the independent or explanatory variable. Since the adjective independent is somewhat mis-leading, although widely used, we shall use the adjective explanatory. Another common term which we shall also use is covariate.

Obviously, not all the father-son pairs of heights lie along the drawn straight line. Equation (10.1) represents the best-fitting straight line of the general form

$$Y = a + b\,X, \tag{10.2}$$

where best-fitting is defined as the unique line which minimizes the average of the squared distances from each observed son's height to the chosen line. More specifically, we write the equation of the best-fitting line as

$$\hat{Y} = \hat{a} + \hat{b}\,X,$$

where $\hat{a}$ and $\hat{b}$ are best choices or estimates for a and b, and $\hat{Y}$ is the value of Y predicted by this model for a specified value of X. In general, statisticians use the ^ notation to indicate that something is an estimate. The line in Figure 10.1 minimizes the average of the values $(Y - \hat{Y})^2$. It is called a linear regression because Y is a straight-line function of the unknown parameters a and b.

Notice that equation (10.1) is an empirical relation, and that it does not imply a causal connection between X and Y.

In this example, the estimated line shows that there is a *regression* of son's heights towards the average. This is indicated by the fact that $\hat{b}$, the multiplier of the father's height, is much less than one. This historical ter-minology has persisted, so that an equation like (10.2) is still called a regres-sion equation, and b is called a *regression coefficient,* whatever its value.

10.3. Multiple Linear Regression

Table 10.1 presents data from an experiment carried out by *Wainwright* et al. [1988] to study nutritional effects on preweaning mouse pups. The level of nutrient availability was manipulated by rearing the pups in litter sizes ranging from three to twelve mice. On day 32, body weight and

Table 10.1. Average weight measurements from 20 litters of mice

Litter size	Body weight, g	Brain weight, g	Litter size	Body weight, g	Brain weight, g
3	9.447	0.444	8	7.040	0.414
3	9.780	0.436	8	7.253	0.409
4	9.155	0.417	9	6.600	0.387
4	9.613	0.429	9	7.260	0.433
5	8.850	0.425	10	6.305	0.410
5	9.610	0.434	10	6.655	0.405
6	8.298	0.404	11	7.183	0.435
6	8.543	0.439	11	6.133	0.407
7	7.400	0.409	12	5.450	0.368
7	8.335	0.429	12	6.050	0.401

brain weight were measured. The values in the table are the average body weight (BODY) and brain weight (W) for each of 20 litters, two of each litter size (LITSIZ). In this study, the effect of nutrition on brain weight is of particular interest.

A simple linear regression model relates a measurement such as brain weight to a single explanatory variable. Equation (10.1) is an example of a simple linear regression model. By comparison, a multiple linear regression model attempts to relate a measurement like brain weight to more than one explanatory variable. If we represent brain weight by W, then a multiple linear regression equation relating W to body weight and litter size would be

$$W = a + b_1(BODY) + b_2(LITSIZ).$$

At this point, it is helpful to introduce a little notation. If Y denotes a response variable and $X_1, X_2, \ldots, X_k$ denote explanatory variables, then a regression equation for Y in terms of $X_1, X_2, \ldots, X_k$ is

$$Y = a + b_1X_1 + b_2X_2 + \ldots + b_kX_k$$

or

$$Y = a + \sum_{i=1}^{k} b_iX_i.$$

Remember, also, that if we wish to refer to specific values of the variables $X_1, X_2, \ldots, X_k$, it is customary to use the lower case letters $x_1, x_2, \ldots, x_k$.

A multiple linear regression analysis finds estimates â, $\hat{b}_1$, ..., $\hat{b}_k$ of a, b_1, ..., b_k which minimize the average value of

$$(Y - \hat{Y})^2 = (Y - \hat{a} - \sum_{i=1}^{k} \hat{b}_i X_i)^2.$$

The assumption which underlies this analysis is that, for specified covariate values $X_1 = x_1$, $X_2 = x_2$, ..., $X_k = x_k$, the distribution of Y is normal with mean or expected value

$$a + \sum_{i=1}^{k} b_i x_i.$$

The variances of the different normal distributions corresponding to different sets of covariate values are assumed to be the same. Notice that a regression analysis makes *no* assumptions about the distribution of the explanatory variables X_1, X_2, ..., X_k.

In our example, two separate, simple linear regressions of brain weight on body weight and litter size can be performed. These lead to the two equations:

$$\hat{W} = 0.336 + 0.010\,(BODY) \text{ and } \hat{W} = 0.447 - 0.004\,(LITSIZ).$$

If the multiplier, or regression coefficient, for any variable was zero, then that variable would have no influence on the dependent variable W. It is very unlikely that the best estimate of a regression coefficient would be exactly zero. A more reasonable question to ask is whether the data provide evidence to contradict the hypothesis that the regression coefficient could be zero, thereby confirming a relationship between the explanatory and dependent variables.

Table 10.2 lists the regression coefficients and their estimated standard errors for the two simple linear regressions of brain weight on body weight and litter size. If there is no relationship between the explanatory variable and brain weight, then it is approximately true that $\hat{b}$, the estimated regression coefficient, is normally distributed with mean zero and variance equal to the square of the estimated standard error. The results of chapter 8, therefore, lead to the test statistic

$$Z = \frac{|\hat{b}|}{\text{est. standard error } (\hat{b})}$$

Table 10.2. Regression coefficients and standard errors for simple linear regressions of brain weight on body weight and litter size

Covariate	Regression coefficient	Estimated standard error	z-statistic	Significance level (p-value)
BODY	0.010	0.002	5.00	<0.0001
LITSIZ	-0.004	0.001	4.00	<0.0001

Table 10.3. Regression coefficients and standard errors for a multiple linear regression of brain weight on body weight and litter size

Covariate	Regression coefficient	Estimated standard error	z-statistic	Significance level (p-value)
BODY	0.024	0.007	3.43	<0.001
LITSIZ	0.007	0.003	2.33	0.020

to test the hypothesis that the regression coefficient b equals zero. To calculate the significance level of the test, the observed value of Z is compared with the critical values of the modulus of a standard normal distribution with mean zero and variance one (cf. Table 8.1). Table 10.2 also includes the observed values of Z and the associated significance levels for each regression coefficient.

Both covariates have very strong relationships with brain weight. The larger the body size, the larger is the brain weight, whereas larger litter sizes are associated with smaller brain weights. Table 10.2 examines the separate effects of body weight and litter size on brain weight. The joint effects of the two variables are investigated via the multiple linear regression equation

$$W = a + b_1(BODY) + b_2(LITSIZ), \tag{10.3}$$

which is estimated by

$$\hat{W} = 0.178 + 0.024(BODY) + 0.007(LITSIZ).$$

Table 10.3 gives the estimated regression coefficients $\hat{b}_1$ and $\hat{b}_2$, their estimated standard errors and the ratios used to test for a non-zero coefficient, based on the model specified by equation (10.3).

Clearly, Table 10.3 is quite different from Table 10.2. The coefficients change in size and, for litter size, in sign. The difference arises because the test for a relationship between LITSIZ, for example, and brain weight in Table 10.3 is performed when the other variable, BODY, is included in the model. Thus, although LITSIZ is inversely related to brain weight when examined singly (see Table 10.2), Table 10.3 tells us that LITSIZ is positively related to brain weight after adjusting for the available information on body weight. On the other hand, body weight is positively related to brain weight, even after litter size is taken into account. Both covariates have coefficients which are significantly different from zero; therefore, each provides information concerning brain weight which is additional to that provided by the other variable. Thus, both covariates should be included in a model describing brain weight.

Table 10.3 is consistent with the biological concept of brain sparing, whereby the nutritional deprivation represented by litter size has a proportionately smaller effect on brain weight than on body weight. In a simple linear regression, litter size is negatively related to brain weight because the larger litters tend to consist of the smaller mice. In the multiple linear regression, the effect of body size is taken into account and the positive regression coefficient associated with litter size indicates that mice from large litters will have larger brain weights than mice of comparable size from smaller litters.

The analysis which we have described in this section is approximate and can be improved upon. The results of a linear regression analysis are frequently presented, in summary form, in an analysis of variance (ANOVA) table. Since this type of presentation does not extend easily to other regression models (see chapters 11 and 12), it is not of primary importance to the aims of this book. Our presentation is consistent with the usual analysis of other regression models which are widely used in medical research, and therefore serves as a useful introduction to the general topic of regression models.

Before we consider other types of regression models, we propose to briefly discuss correlation analysis, a historical antecedent to regression analysis. Also, the final section of this chapter describes ANOVA tables. This material is not needed to understand chapters 11 and 12, but is included for completeness. The amount of detail which is necessary to explain ANOVA tables far exceeds the complexity of any other explanation appearing in this book. We therefore suggest that the reader bypass § 10.5 on a first reading.

10.4. Correlation

Regression models presuppose there is an outcome variable of some importance, and that interest in other variables derives from their potential influence on the outcome variable. Historically, the development of regression analysis was preceded by another approach known as correlation analysis.

Consider the case of two variables, Y and X. In a regression analysis, we assume Y has a normal distribution, but X may take any value and no distributional assumptions about X are required. Thus, X may be determined along with Y, X values may be fixed by the experimenter, e.g., X represents treatment received in a randomized clinical trial, or any number of factors might influence the X values observed in the data. Correlation analysis is restricted to the situation when X and Y are both random variables, and commonly assumes that both variables have a normal distribution.

Figure 10.2 shows separate plots of brain weight versus litter size and body weight, and litter size versus body weight. The plots indicate that when brain weight is high or low, body weight tends to be correspondingly high or low, whereas litter size tends to be the opposite. The relationship between litter size and body weight is similar to the relationship between brain weight and litter size. A numerical measure of the observed association between two variables is the correlation coefficient r. For completeness, we give the formula for r, which is

$$r = \frac{\sum_{i=1}^{n} (x_i - \bar{x})(y_i - \bar{y})}{\sqrt{\sum_{i=1}^{n} (x_i - \bar{x})^2 \sum_{i=1}^{n} (y_i - \bar{y})^2}},$$

where n is the number of paired observations on X and Y.

The correlation coefficient is a number between -1 and 1; the value $r = 0$ indicates there is no linear relationship between the two variables. A statistical procedure has been developed to test the hypothesis of no association between X and Y, based on the observed correlation coefficient, but we do not intend to discuss it here. If r is negative, then X and Y are said to be negatively correlated, implying that low values of X tend to occur with high values of Y and vice-versa. This kind of association is illustrated by the relationship between brain weight and litter size, which have a correlation

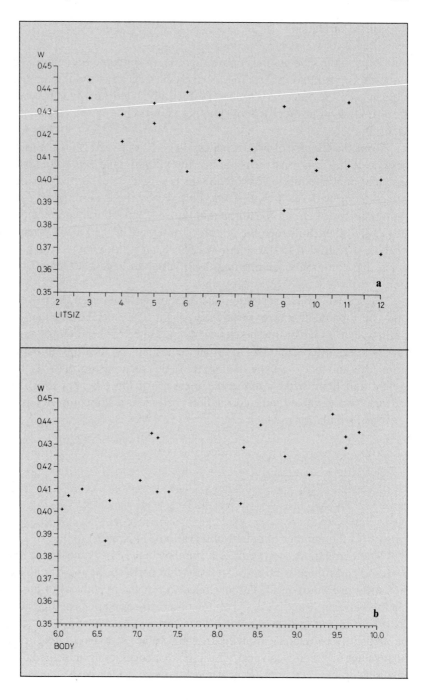

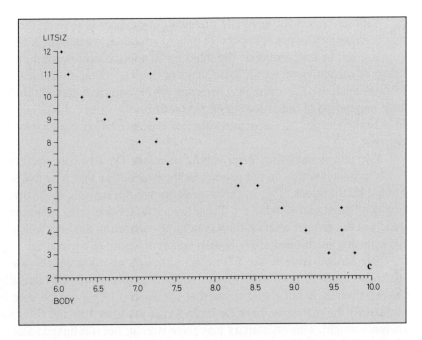

Fig. 10.2. Scatterplots of average weight measurements from 20 litters of mice. **a** Brain weight (W) vs. litter size (LITSIZ). **b** W vs. body weight (BODY). **c** LITSIZ vs. BODY.

coefficient of −0.62. If r is positive, then X and Y have a relationship like that observed between brain weight and body weight. The correlation coefficient for these variables is 0.75.

The correlation coefficient can be used in the initial examination of a data set to identify relationships which deserve further study. However, it is generally more useful to think of linking two variables via a regression equation. From a regression analysis we can see very directly how changes in one variable are associated with changes in the other outcome variable. The regressions of litter size on brain weight and body weight are summarized by the equations:

$$\widehat{\text{LITSIZ}} = 47.41 - 95.76(W) \text{ and } \widehat{\text{LITSIZ}} = 23.51 - 2.07(\text{BODY}).$$

Thus, for a specified value of brain weight or body weight, we could 'predict' a value for litter size.

Another reason for generally preferring regression analysis is the fact that correlation analysis is applicable only to situations when both X and Y are random. In many studies, the selection of subjects will depend on the values of certain variables for these subjects. Such selection invalidates correlation analysis. For example, *Armitage* [1971] indicates that if, from a large population of individuals, selection restricts the values of one variable to a limited range, the absolute value of the correlation coefficient will decrease.

Two additional points deserve brief mention. The first concerns correlation measures which do not depend on the assumption that X and Y have normal distributions. Two of these measures are Spearman's rank correlation coefficient and Kendall's τ. These are useful for analyzing non-normal data, but the general reservations concerning correlation analysis which we have already mentioned apply equally to any measure of correlation.

The second issue is the following. Although we advocate the use of regression models, it is important to realize that the estimated regression line of Y on X is not the same as that for X on Y. This can be seen by comparing the regression lines for brain weight on litter size and litter size on brain weight. This asymmetry may seem strange, but it is linked to use of the differences $(Y - \hat{Y})$ as an estimation criterion. If one variable is random, say Y, and the other is selectively sampled, then the regression of Y on X will be sensible. Otherwise, the choice of a suitable regression model may be determined by some preference for predicting one variable on the basis of the other.

10.5. The Analysis of Variance

As we mentioned in § 10.3, a multiple regression analysis is frequently summarized in an analysis of variance (ANOVA) table. This section, which is not necessary to the understanding of any subsequent material, provides a brief introduction to ANOVA tables. On a first reading, we strongly advise that the reader omit this section and proceed to chapter 11.

In the example we have been discussing, we have observed values of the response variable, W, and predicted values, $\hat{W}$, which are derived from the regression equation. Let $\overline{W}$ represent the average of all the observed brain weights. In chapter 1, we learned that measures of spread, such as variance, usually involve the quantity $(W - \overline{W})$, which represents the difference of observed values of W from their average. Strictly speaking, we should refer to $(W - \overline{W})^2$ rather than the simple difference $(W - \overline{W})$. We will shortly introduce the squared difference; however, it is simpler, for the moment, to begin our explanation by discussing $(W - \overline{W})$. In fact, the analysis of variance is based on the relation

$$(W - \overline{W}) = (W - \hat{W}) + (\hat{W} - \overline{W}),$$

which decomposes $(W - \overline{W})$ into two separate components. If we regard $(W - \overline{W})$ as 'total variation', i.e., variance, it is natural to ask what components of variation $(W - \hat{W})$ and $(\hat{W} - \overline{W})$ represent.

In the absence of a regression model for the mean value of W, the dependent variable, $\overline{W}$ represents a natural estimate. Thus, $(W - \overline{W})$ can be interpreted as the variation of W around this natural estimate. Once we have specified a regression model for the mean value of W, we have a different estimate, $\hat{W}$, which is based on the model. Moreover, $(W - \hat{W})$ will generally be smaller than $(W - \overline{W})$. Therefore, of the total variation represented by $(W - \overline{W})$, the component $(\hat{W} - \overline{W})$ has been 'explained' or accounted for by the fitted regression model for W. That is, since $\hat{W}$ is now the estimated mean value of W, based on the values of LITSIZ and BODY, we expect to see W differ from $\overline{W}$ by $(\hat{W} - \overline{W})$. The remaining component, $(W - \hat{W})$, is called the 'residual variation', i.e., the variation in W which is not explained by the regression equation.

Now that we have informally described the decomposition of the variance in W, we introduce squared differences, which are the correct representation. Let W_1, W_2, ..., W_n be n observed values of W, and let $\overline{W} = \frac{1}{n} \sum_{i=1}^{n} W_i$ be their average. The total variation in these data can be represented by

$$\sum_{i=1}^{n} (W_i - \overline{W})^2 = (W_1 - \overline{W})^2 + (W_2 - \overline{W})^2 + \ldots + (W_n - \overline{W})^2,$$

which is $(n - 1)$ times the sample variance for W. Although it is not obvious, it can be shown that

$$\sum_{i=1}^{n} (W_i - \overline{W})^2 = \sum_{i=1}^{n} (W_i - \hat{W}_i)^2 + \sum_{i=1}^{n} (\hat{W}_i - \overline{W})^2.$$

Thus, the total variation in W decomposes into two sums of squared differences. In view of the preceding discussion involving simple differences, it should not be difficult to accept that the second sum represents the component of total variation in W which is accounted for by the fitted regression model, while the first sum represents the residual variation. If we use SS to represent a sum of squares, then we can rewrite the above equation, symbolically, as

$$SS_{Total} = SS_{Residual} + SS_{Regression};$$

the reasons for the subscripts should be quite obvious.

Each sum of squares of the form

$$\sum_{i=1}^{n} (W_i - [\text{estimated value of } W_i])^2$$

has associated with it a quantity called its degrees of freedom (DF). This quantity is equal to the number of terms in the sum minus the number of values which must be calculated from the W_i's in order to specify all the estimated values. For example, in SS_{Total} the estimated value for each W_i is the same, namely $\overline{W}$. Thus, we need one calculated value, and the degrees of freedom for SS_{Total} are $(n-1)$. For $SS_{Residual}$, the estimated value of each W_i is equal to

$$\hat{W}_i = \hat{a} + \sum_{j=1}^{k} \hat{b}_j x_j,$$

where $x_1, \ldots, x_k$ are the values of the covariates corresponding to W_i. These n estimates require $(k+1)$ calculated values, $\hat{a}, \hat{b}_1, \ldots, \hat{b}_k$; therefore, the degrees of freedom for $SS_{Residual}$ are $(n-k-1)$.

Although we shall not attempt to justify the following result, it can be shown that

$$DF_{Total} = DF_{Residual} + DF_{Regression}.$$

Therefore, since DF_{Total} equals $(n-1)$ and $DF_{Residual}$ equals $(n-k-1)$, it follows that the degrees of freedom for $SS_{Regression}$ are equal to k.

The only remaining unknown quantities which appear in an ANOVA table are called mean squares (MS); these are defined to be the ratio of a sum of squares to its degrees of freedom, i.e., MS = SS/DF. The variance estimates which we discussed in chapter 9 can be recognized as mean squares, and this is partly the reason that statisticians call the method of analysis which we are presently describing 'the analysis of variance'.

Table 10.4. ANOVA table for the regression analysis of brain weight

Term	SS ($\times 10^{-5}$)	DF	MS ($\times 10^{-5}$)	F
Regression	452.1	2	226.1	15.8
Residual	242.9	17	14.3	
Total	695.0	19		

$R^2 = 0.65$.

The typical format for an ANOVA table is shown in Table 10.4, which gives the appropriate entries for the regression of W on BODY and LITSIZ. From this table, two quantities are usually calculated. The first of these is a ratio called R^2 (R-squared), which is equal to

$$R^2 = SS_{Regression}/SS_{Total}.$$

This ratio indicates the fraction of the total variation in W which is accounted for by the fitted regression model. There are no formal statistical tests associated with R^2, and it is primarily used for information purposes only. In Table 10.4, the value of R^2 is 0.65, indicating that 65% of the total variation in W is explained by the regression model.

The second quantity which is calculated from an ANOVA table such as Table 10.4 is the ratio of $MS_{Regression}$ to $MS_{Residual}$. This number is frequently called an F-ratio because, if the null hypothesis that *all* the regression coefficients $b_1, \ldots, b_k$ are equal to zero is true, the ratio $MS_{Regression}/MS_{Residual}$ should have an F-distribution with $DF_{Regression}$ and $DF_{Residual}$ degrees of freedom. Recall that the F-distribution was introduced in §9.5.

The observed value of this F-ratio is usually compared with the critical values for the appropriate F-distribution (see Table 9.7), and if the observed value exceeds the critical value, the regression is said to be significant, i.e., the data contradict the null hypothesis that all the regression coefficients are zero. In Table 10.4, the observed F-ratio is 226.1/14.3 = 15.8. Since the 5% critical value for an F-distribution with 2 and 17 degrees of freedom is 3.59, we conclude that the regression is significant at the 5% level; the data contradict the hypothesis that both BODY and LITSIZ have no effect on brain weight. This result is consistent with the conclusion which we reached in

Table 10.5. An expanded ANOVA table for the regression analysis of brain weight

Term	SS ($\times 10^{-5}$)		DF	MS ($\times 10^{-5}$)	F
Regression	452.1		2	226.1	15.8
BODY		386.9	1	386.9	27.1
LITSIZ|BODY		65.2	1	65.2	4.6
Residual	242.9		17	14.3	
Total	695.0		19		

§ 10.3 (cf. Table 10.3) that the regression coefficients for BODY and LITSIZ are significantly different from zero.

Table 10.3 summarizes the results of tests concerning the effect of individual covariates when the other covariate was included in the regression model. For example, we determined whether LITSIZ had any influence on brain weight if BODY was already included in the model. By comparison, the F-test which we have discussed above is a joint test of the hypothesis that all the regression coefficients are zero. However, the ANOVA table which we have described can be generalized to address the question of the individual effect of each covariate.

If we had calculated an ANOVA table for the regression of W on BODY, then the $SS_{Regression}$ would have been 386.9×10^{-5}, and $DF_{Regression}$ would have been one. This number, 386.9×10^{-5}, represents the component of the $SS_{Regression}$ in Table 10.4 which is due to BODY alone. If we next add LITSIZ to the regression equation, so that we are fitting the model described by Table 10.4, the $SS_{Regression}$ increases by 65.2×10^{-5}, from 386.9×10^{-5} to 452.1×10^{-5}. Thus, 65.2×10^{-5} is the component of $SS_{Regression}$ which is accounted for by LITSIZ, when the model already includes BODY. Notice, also, that we could have performed these calculations in the reverse order, i.e., LITSIZ first, followed by BODY.

In Table 10.5, the $SS_{Regression}$ is divided into two parts. One part is labelled BODY, and represents the component of $SS_{Regression}$ which is due to BODY; the other part is labelled LITSIZ|BODY, and represents the component which is due to LITSIZ in addition to BODY. The degrees of freedom for each component in the sum of squares are one since $DF_{Regression}$ equals two and the component of the $SS_{Regression}$ which is due to BODY has one degree of freedom. Therefore, two F-ratios can be calculated, and these

Table 10.6. An ANOVA table for the regression of brain weight on litter size

Term	SS ($\times 10^{-5}$)	DF	MS ($\times 10^{-5}$)	F
Regression	268.4	1	268.4	11.32
Residual	426.6	18	23.7	
Lack of Fit	129.0	8	16.1	0.54
Pure Error	297.6	10	9.8	
Total	695.0	19		

appear in the last column of Table 10.5; one F-ratio corresponds to BODY alone, and the other represents LITSIZ|BODY. If the null hypothesis that BODY has no influence on W is true, the F-ratio for BODY should have an F-distribution on 1 and 17 degrees of freedom. Quite separately, if the null hypothesis is true that LITSIZ has no influence on W which is additional to the effect of BODY, then the F-ratio for LITSIZ|BODY should also have an F-distribution on 1 and 17 degrees of freedom. Since the 5% critical value for this particular F-distribution is 4.45, we conclude that each of the terms in the regression model – BODY and LITSIZ|BODY – is necessary since a test of the respective null hypothesis has a significance level of less than 5%. This conclusion coincides with the analysis which we discussed in § 10.3 (cf. Table 10.3).

To illustrate one additional type of calculation, Table 10.6 presents an ANOVA table for the simple linear regression of brain weight on litter size. We assume no additional variables are available. In an analysis of variance, the $MS_{Residual}$ is often used as an estimate of variance. The $MS_{Residual}$ represents the variation which cannot be accounted for by the regression equation, and it is often assumed that this unexplained variation is the natural variance of the observations about the estimated values which are determined by the regression equation. Since we have two independent observations on each of the ten litter sizes, we can calculate a separate, independent estimate of the natural variation in the model. Let W_1 and W_2 represent the two observations for a single litter size. The natural estimate of the mean brain weight for this litter size is $\overline{W} = (W_1 + W_2)/2$, and an estimate of the residual variation, based on these weights alone, would be a SS which is equal to $(W_1 - \overline{W})^2 + (W_2 - \overline{W})^2$. Since we have two terms in the sum and one estimate, $\overline{W}$, the degrees of freedom for this sum would be two. If we repeat this calculation for all ten litter sizes, then the total of the ten individual sums of squares is 297.6×10^{-5}, and this total sum of squares would have $10 \times 1 = 10$ degrees of freedom.

This type of calculation, which leads to a MS of $297.6 \times 10^{-5}/10 = 29.8 \times 10^{-5}$ in our example, is often called a calculation of 'pure error'. This is because, regardless of the information we have concerning an individual litter size, the variation of independent observations from litters of the same size can never be accounted for by the regression equation. Therefore, $MS_{Pure\ Error}$ is a better estimate of the natural variance of the observations than $MS_{Residual}$. Recall that we are assuming we do not have any information apart from brain weight and litter size. To calculate a $SS_{Pure\ Error}$ for the regression summarized in Table 10.5 would require independent observations on mice which have the same body weight and were reared in litters of the same size. Such observations are not available, and therefore the pure error calculations cannot be carried out in that particular case.

The $SS_{Pure\ Error}$ is one component of $SS_{Residual}$, and the remainder is usually called the Lack of Fit component, since it constitutes a part of the SS_{Total} which cannot be accounted for, either by the regression model or by pure error. The $SS_{Lack\ of\ Fit}$ measures the potential for improvement in the model for W if additional covariate information is used, or possibly if an alternative form of the regression equation is specified instead of the current version. A test that the lack of fit in the current model is significant can be based on the F-ratio $MS_{Lack\ of\ Fit}/MS_{Pure\ Error}$. If the null hypothesis that there is no lack of fit in the current model is true, this ratio should have an F-distribution with degrees of freedom $DF_{Lack\ of\ Fit} = DF_{Residual} - DF_{Pure\ Error}$ and $DF_{Pure\ Error}$. We will not discuss the question of lack of fit in detail; however, if there is a significant lack of fit, it is customary to plot the values of $W - \hat{W}$ for all the observations, to see if they appear to be normally distributed. If so, then the lack of fit is usually attributed to unavailable information rather than the existence of better alternative models which involve the same variates. In Table 10.6, the test for Lack of Fit is not significant.

If the Lack of Fit component of $SS_{Residual}$ is significant, then sometimes $MS_{Pure\ Error}$ is used as the denominator in the F-ratios for $SS_{Regression}$ and its components. This is advisable if the degrees of freedom associated with $MS_{Pure\ Error}$ are reasonably large. In general, the use of $MS_{Residual}$ will be more conservative. When the Lack of Fit component is not significant, it is appropriate to use $MS_{Residual}$, and we have done this in calculating the regression F-ratio shown in Table 10.6.

11 Binary Logistic Regression

11.1. Introduction

One reason that linear regression is not as widely used in medical statistics as in other fields is that the outcome variable in a medical study frequently cannot be assumed to have a normal distribution. A common type of response or outcome variable in medical research is a binary variable. These response variables take one of two values, and were discussed extensively in chapters 2 through 5. In this chapter, we describe a particular regression model for a binary response variable.

To illustrate the methodology, we shall consider an example concerning bone marrow transplantation for the treatment of aplastic anemia. One response of major interest is graft rejection. A binary variable, Y, can be defined so that Y = 1 corresponds to graft rejection and Y = 0 represents graft acceptance.

Table 11.1 is taken from an article by *Storb* et al. [1977]. It presents a binary logistic regression analysis of graft rejection, relating the response variable, Y, to marrow cell dose in units of 10^8 cells per kilogram of body weight, patient age in decades, extent of prior blood units transfused, transplant year (minus 1970) and preceding androgen treatment. The prior blood

Table 11.1. Maximum likelihood fit of a binary logistic regression model to marrow-graft rejection data on 68 patients with aplastic anemia [*Storb* et al., 1977]

Factor	Logistic coefficient	Standard error	Ratio
Marrow cell dose	−1.005	0.344	−2.92 (p < 0.01)
Age	−0.457	0.275	−1.66 (p < 0.10)
Blood units	1.112	0.672	1.65 (p < 0.10)
Transplant year	0.735	0.319	2.30 (p < 0.05)
Androgen treatment	1.417	0.805	1.76 (p < 0.10)

Reprinted, by permission of The New England Journal of Medicine *296:* 64 (1977).

unit variable was zero if the patient received less than 10 whole blood units prior to transplantation, and one otherwise. The androgen variable was zero if the patient had not received androgen previously, and one otherwise. Let us call these five variables X_1, X_2, X_3, X_4, and X_5. A convenient, shorthand notation for the set of variables $\{X_1, X_2, X_3, X_4, X_5\}$ is $\underline{X}$. Remember, also, that we denote a particular value for a variable by the corresponding lower case letter, viz $\underline{x} = \{x_1, x_2, x_3, x_4, x_5\}$.

11.2. Logistic Regression

Since Y can assume only two possible values, it would be unrealistic to entertain a linear regression model such as

$$Y = a + b_1X_1 + \ldots + b_5X_5 = a + \sum_{i=1}^{5} b_iX_i.$$

Theoretically, the right-hand side of this equation can take any value between minus infinity $(-\infty)$ and plus infinity $(+\infty)$ unless we restrict the values of a and the regression coefficients $b_1, \ldots, b_5$.

In a linear regression model, the expression $a + \sum b_iX_i$ is assumed to be the expected value of a normal distribution. The expected value of a binary variable such as Y turns out to be the probability that $Y = 1$. Thus, it is more reasonable to consider a regression model which involves the probability of graft rejection, i.e., $Pr(Y = 1)$. A probability lies between zero and one, and this is still too narrow a range of values for the expression $a + \sum b_iX_i$. However, if a probability, say p, is between 0 and 1, then $p/(1-p)$ belongs to the interval $(0, \infty)$ and $\log\{p/(1-p)\}$ belongs to the interval $(-\infty, \infty)$. This is the same range of values to which the expression $a + \sum b_iX_i$ belongs.

If we represent the probability of graft rejection, $Y = 1$, by $Pr(Y = 1 | \underline{x})$ for an individual with covariate values $\underline{x}$, then a binary logistic regression model for Y is specified by the equation

$$\log\left\{\frac{Pr(Y = 1 | \underline{x})}{1 - Pr(Y = 1 | \underline{x})}\right\} = \log\left\{\frac{Pr(Y = 1 | \underline{x})}{Pr(Y = 0 | \underline{x})}\right\} = a + \sum_{i=1}^{5} b_iX_i.$$

An equivalent way of specifying the model is via the equation

$$Pr(Y = 1 | \underline{x}) = \frac{\exp(a + \sum_{i=1}^{5} b_ix_i)}{1 + \exp(a + \sum_{i=1}^{5} b_ix_i)},$$

which reveals that the model links the linear expression $a + \Sigma\, b_i x_i$ to the probability of graft rejection. Now, as in linear regression, if b_i is zero, then the factor represented by X_i is not associated with graft rejection. As in the case of linear regression analysis (see chapter 10), a suitable statistic for testing the hypothesis that the regression coefficient, b_i, equals zero is

$$Z = \frac{|\hat{b}_i|}{\text{est. standard error } (\hat{b}_i)}\ .$$

Occasionally, the results of an analysis may be presented in terms of the ratio

$$\frac{\hat{b}_i}{\text{est. standard error } (\hat{b}_i)},$$

which is equal to Z, apart from the sign. This is the situation in Table 11.1. In either case, the conclusion regarding the covariate represented by X_i is the same.

In Table 11.1, the largest ratio is associated with marrow cell dose ($p = 0.004$). Transplant year has a significant effect on graft rejection, with a p-value of 0.02. The other covariates are not significant at the 5% level, although the associated p-values are all less than 0.10. Remember that a test of the hypothesis that a certain regression coefficient is zero is a test for the importance of the corresponding covariate, having adjusted for all the other variables in the regression model. For example, the effect of transplant year cannot be attributed to a change in marrow cell dose values with time, since marrow cell dose is included in the model when we test the hypothesis $b_4 = 0$, i.e., the covariate representing transplant year is not associated with graft rejection.

Details of the calculations which are involved in estimating a binary logistic regression model are beyond the scope of this book. To actually use this methodology to analyze a particular set of data, it would be necessary to consult a statistician. However, we hope our brief discussion of the binary logistic regression model has been informative, and will permit readers to critically appraise the use of this technique in published papers.

There are many aspects which are common to the use of quite different regression models. For this reason, we have minimized our discussion of binary logistic regression; much of the discussion in chapter 12 is equally relevant to logistic regression. Nevertheless, as another illustration of this methodology, and as a means of addressing a topic which we have thus far neglected, we discuss the application of logistic regression to 2×2 tables in the next section.

Table 11.2. Graft rejection status and marrow cell dose data for 68 aplastic anemia patients

Graft rejection	Marrow cell dose (10^8 cells/kg)		Total
	< 3.0	≥ 3.0	
Yes	17	4	21
No	19	28	47
Total	36	32	68

Table 11.3. A logistic regression analysis of graft rejection and marrow cell dose in 68 aplastic anemia patients

Coefficient	Estimate	Estimated standard error	z-statistic
a	−1.95	0.53	–
b	1.84	0.63	2.92 (p = 0.004)

11.3. Estimation in 2 × 2 Tables

The discussion of 2 × 2 tables in chapters 2 through 5 concentrates on the concept of a significance test. This emphasis was adopted for pedagogical purposes, and we now turn to the equally important problem of estimation in 2 × 2 tables. This can be done within the framework of the binary logistic regression model.

Consider the data presented in Table 11.2 concerning graft rejection in 68 aplastic anemia patients; each marrow cell dose is recorded as being one of two types, namely either less than or at least 3.0×10^8 cells/kg. Let Y represent graft rejection as in §§11.1, 11.2 and let X be a binary covariate, where X = 1 corresponds to a low marrow cell dose and X = 0 indicates a higher dose. A binary logistic regression model for graft rejection and marrow cell dose is specified by the equation

$$\Pr(Y = 1 \mid x) = \frac{\exp(a + bx)}{1 + \exp(a + bx)}. \tag{11.1}$$

Therefore, the probability of graft rejection for a high marrow cell dose
(X = 0) is exp(a)/{1 + exp(a)}; the corresponding probability for the lower dose
(X = 1) is exp(a + b)/{1 + exp(a + b)}.

The estimation of b is of major importance in studying the influence of
marrow cell dose on graft rejection. Table 11.3 presents the estimation of
model (11.1) for the data in Table 11.2. A test of the hypothesis that b, the
regression coefficient, equals zero is based on the observed value of the test
statistic $Z = |\hat{b}|/\{$est. standard error$(\hat{b})\}$ which equals 2.92. Since this observed
value exceeds the 5% critical point given in Table 8.1, there is evidence to
contradict the hypothesis that marrow cell dose does not influence graft
rejection, i.e., the hypothesis that b equals zero.

The larger $\hat{b}$ is, the larger is the estimated effect of a low marrow cell dose
on graft rejection. As we saw in chapter 8, $\hat{b}$ is only a single number, and if we
wish to estimate b, a confidence interval should also be calculated. A 95%
confidence interval for b is defined to be

$$\hat{b} \pm 1.96\{\text{est. standard error } (\hat{b})\},$$

and can be represented by the interval (b_L, b_H).

The simplest way to think about b is in terms of an odds ratio. If p
represents the probability of graft rejection, then p/(1 − p) is called the odds in
favor of rejection. Now, let p_1 represent the probability of rejection for the
higher marrow cell dose and p_2 the corresponding probability for the lower
dose; then the ratio

$$\frac{p_2/(1-p_2)}{p_1/(1-p_1)}$$

is called the odds ratio (OR). If equation (11.1) is used to define p_1 and p_2,
then it turns out that

$$OR = e^b.$$

Since a 95% confidence interval for b is (b_L, b_H), the corresponding interval
for the odds ratio, OR, is

$$(e^{b_L}, e^{b_H}),$$

with an estimate of OR being $\widehat{OR} = \exp(\hat{b})$.

For a simple 2 × 2 table, the formula for $\hat{b}$ can be stated explicitly. If the
table is of the form shown in Table 11.4, then

$$\hat{b} = \log\left(\frac{ad}{bc}\right) \quad \text{and} \quad \widehat{OR} = \frac{ad}{bc}.$$

Table 11.4. The format of a 2 × 2 table in which the estimate of the odds ratio is ad/bc; the symbols – and + indicate absence and presence, respectively

Factor 2	Factor 1	
	–	+
–	a	b
+	c	d

Table 11.5. Graft rejection and marrow cell dose data in 68 aplastic anemia patients stratified by year of transplant

Graft rejection	Transplant year after 1972					
	no marrow cell dose (10^8 cells/kg)			yes marrow cell dose (10^8 cells/kg)		
	<3.0	$\geqslant 3.0$	total	<3.0	$\geqslant 3.0$	total
Yes	4	2	6	13	2	15
No	9	16	25	10	12	22
Total	13	18	31	23	14	37
	Table 1			Table 2		

In addition, an approximation to the estimated standard error of $\hat{b}$, based on the logistic regression model, is

$$\left(\frac{1}{a} + \frac{1}{b} + \frac{1}{c} + \frac{1}{d}\right)^{1/2}.$$

This estimate can be somewhat too small, but it is convenient for quick calculation. In our example, the approximate value is 0.63, which is equal to the estimate of 0.63 from the logistic regression analysis.

In chapter 5, we discussed the use of stratification to adjust the test for no association in a 2 × 2 table for possible heterogeneity in the study population. In general, regression models are designed to make such adjustments

Table 11.6. A logistic regression analysis of graft rejection and marrow cell dose, stratified by year of transplant

Coefficient	Estimate	Estimated standard error	z-statistic
a_1	-2.37	0.65	–
a_2	-1.54	0.59	–
b	1.72	0.64	2.69 (p = 0.007)

more efficiently, but the stratification approach can be viewed as a special case of a regression model.

In the regression model for graft rejection, represented by the equation

$$Pr(Y = 1 \mid x) = \frac{\exp(a + bx)}{1 + \exp(a + bx)},$$

the parameter a determines the probability of graft rejection in individuals with $X = 0$, while b measures the change in this probability if $X = 1$. Other factors relevant to graft rejection would alter the overall probability of rejection in subgroups of the data. For example, Table 11.2 can be subdivided into two 2×2 tables by stratifying according to transplant year (After 1972 – No or Yes). This is done in Table 11.5. If these two tables are numbered 1 and 2, then we would define the two logistic regression models

$$Pr(Y = 1 \mid x) = \begin{cases} \dfrac{\exp(a_1 + bx)}{1 + \exp(a_1 + bx)} & \text{for Table 1,} \\[3mm] \dfrac{\exp(a_2 + bx)}{1 + \exp(a_2 + bx)} & \text{for Table 2.} \end{cases} \tag{11.2}$$

In these models, the probability of rejection changes from Table 1 to Table 2 because the parameter a varies; however, the odds ratio parameter b, which measures the association between marrow cell dose and graft rejection, does not change. This type of model underlies the approach to combining 2×2 tables which we described in chapter 5. For any subclassifications of the population, including matched pairs, we can specify logistic regression models for each subgroup by using different a parameters and the same b parameter. Based on these models, b is estimated in order to study the association of interest.

Table 11.6 presents the estimation of model (11.2). The estimate of $\hat{b}$ is 1.72 and the observed value of the statistic used to test for no association is 1.72/0.64 = 2.69. This result is consistent with the unstratified analysis which we discussed earlier.

Table 11.6 also records estimates of a_1 and a_2. As the number of subgroups becomes large, problems do arise in estimating the a parameters. Specialized methodology for estimating b, alone, does exist and should be used in these situations; however, the details of this methodology are beyond the scope of this book. For our purposes, the nature of the logistic regression model, and the use of $\hat{b}$ to test for association, are more important.

Finally, we note that it is possible to test the assumption that the odds ratio, exp(b), is the same in the stratified 2×2 tables. If there are only a few tables, we can calculate separate interval estimates of b for each table and see if they overlap. More formal tests are rather complicated, but should be carried out if the assumption that b is constant is thought to be questionable in the least. A statistician should be consulted concerning these tests, and the appropriate way to proceed with the analysis, if the assumption that b is the same in the stratified 2×2 tables is not supported by the data.

Comment:

Readers who dip into the epidemiological literature will observe that logistic regression is being used increasingly to analyze case-control studies. In this literature, it is common to see exp(b) referred to as a relative risk. For the model defined in equation (11.1), the relative risk associated with a low marrow cell dose would be $Pr(Y = 1 \mid X = 1)/ Pr(Y = 1 \mid X = 0)$, or p_2/p_1 in our later notation. For a rare disease, the type usually investigated via a case-control study, p_1 and p_2 are small and therefore $1 - p_1$ and $1 - p_2$ are close to 1. In this situation, there is little difference between the odds ratio $\{p_2/(1 - p_2)\}/\{p_1/(1 - p_1)\}$ and the relative risk p_2/p_1. Therefore, epidemiologists frequently ignore the approximation which is involved, and refer to estimates of odds ratios from a case-control study as estimates of relative risks. In §16.4 we discuss the use of logistic regression models in the analysis of case-control data. It is worth noting that this particular application of logistic regression involves certain arguments which go beyond the scope of this book. However, the nature of the conclusions arising from such an approach will be as we have presented them in this chapter.

Table 11.7. Data from a study of fetal mortality and prenatal care (L≡Less, M≡More) in two clinics

Prenatal care	Clinic 1		Clinic 2	
	L	M	L	M
Died	12	16	34	4
Survived	176	293	197	23

Table 11.8. Two logistic regression analyses of fetal mortality and prenatal care

	Coefficient	Estimate	Estimated standard error	z-statistic
Unstratified	a	−2.76	0.23	–
model	b	0.67	0.28	2.39 (p = 0.017)
Stratified	a_1	−2.88	0.24	–
model	a_2	−1.89	0.35	–
	b	0.15	0.33	0.45 (p = 0.65)

11.4. Reanalysis of a Previous Example

In chapter 5, we discussed data concerning fetal mortality and prenatal care (L = less, M≡ more) in two clinics. The data are summarized in the 2×2 tables shown in Table 11.7. Logistic regression analyses of these data, based on the unstratified model (see equation 11.1) and the stratified model (see equation 11.2), are given in Table 11.8. As we found in chapter 5, the unstratified model indicates there is a significant association (p = 0.017), whereas the more appropriate stratified analysis suggests that there is no association (p = 0.65) between fetal mortality and the amount of prenatal care received.

Tables 11.3, 11.6 and 11.8 illustrate that a stratified analysis, although generally appropriate, may or may not lead to different conclusions than an unstratified analysis. It is the potential for different conclusions that makes the adjustment for heterogeneity in a population important.

11.5. The Analysis of Dose-Response Data

As we have already seen in previous sections of this chapter, the binary logistic regression model is ideal for analyzing the dependence of a binary response variable on a set of explanatory variables, or covariates. Therefore, we wish to emphasize that the method of analysis which is discussed in this section is simply a special case of binary logistic regression. However, it represents a situation that is common in clinical studies. Moreover, the clinical example which we intend to discuss involves certain aspects of regression models which have not arisen in any of the examples we have previously considered.

Duncan et al. [1984] report the results of a study which was initiated to investigate the effect of premedication on the dose requirement in children of the anaesthetic thiopentone. The study involved observations on 490 children aged 1–12 years. These patients were divided into four groups, three of which received different types of premedication. No premedication of any kind was administered to the fourth group of patients. All the children subsequently received an injection of 2.0–8.5 mg/kg of thiopentone in steps of 0.5 mg/kg. The anaesthetic was administered to each patient over a 10-second interval, and the eyelash reflex was tested 20 seconds after the end of the thiopentone injection. If the eyelash reflex was abolished, the patient was deemed to have responded to the anaesthetic.

The investigation described above is typical of a class of clinical studies involving a binary response variable. Clearly, the purpose of the research is to assess the dependence of the response on a continuous variable which is under the control of the researcher. Investigations of this type are generally referred to as dose-response studies, because the clinician administers a measured concentration of a particular substance to each subject in a sample and then observes whether or not the subject exhibits the designated response. A principal assumption on which dose-response studies are based is the notion that the probability of responding depends in a simple, smooth way on the concentration. Figure 11.1 shows an example of this smooth relationship. In addition to estimating this dependence, researchers are usually interested in questions which concern differences in the dependence on concentration among well-defined subgroups of the population.

The method of binary logistic regression, which we introduced in §§11.1 and 11.2, is ideally suited to the analysis of dose-response data. In the use of this regression model to analyze data from such a study, it is

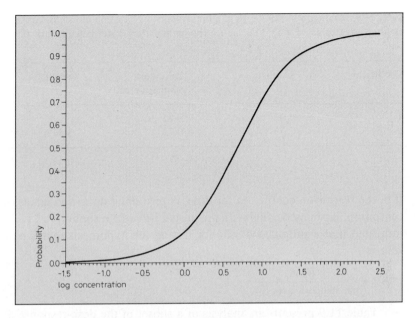

Fig. 11.1. A graph showing how the probability of responding might depend on the logarithm of the concentration in a dose-response study.

common practice to choose the logarithm of the measured concentration as the explanatory variable rather than the actual concentration. Since use of the logarithmic value tends to improve the fit of the model to the data, we will follow this convention and represent the log concentration, or dose, of the administered substance by the letter d.

Let the binary variable Y denote the observed response, with $Y = 1$ indicating occurrence of the event of interest and $Y = 0$ its absence. Then $Pr(Y = 1 | d)$ represents the probability of observing the designated response in a subject who receives dose d. As we saw in §11.2, a binary logistic regression model for Y is specified by the equation

$$\log\left\{\frac{Pr(Y = 1 | d)}{1 - Pr(Y = 1 | d)}\right\} = \log\left\{\frac{Pr(Y = 1 | d)}{Pr(Y = 0 | d)}\right\} = a + bd,$$

which is equivalent to requiring that

$$Pr(Y = 1 | d) = \frac{e^{a + bd}}{1 + e^{a + bd}}.$$

Table 11.9. Maximum likelihood fit of a binary logistic regression model to data on 137 children premedicated with TDP and atropine and then anaesthetized with thiopentone

Coefficient	Estimate	Estimated standard error	z-statistic
a	−1.92	0.82	−
b	2.78	0.72	3.86 (p = 0.0001)

If b, the regression coefficient for dose, is zero, then dose, and hence concentration, is not associated with the probability of a response. In §11.2 we indicated that a suitable statistic for testing the hypothesis that b equals zero is

$$Z = \frac{|\hat{b}|}{\text{est. standard error } (\hat{b})} .$$

Table 11.9 presents an analysis of a subset of the dose-response data which were collected for the study described by *Duncan* et al. [1984]. The data were made available by Mr. *B. Newman.* The results summarized in the table pertain solely to the group of 137 patients who were premedicated orally with TDP (trimeprazine, droperiodol and physeptone) and atropine. As we might expect, the regression analysis shows that dose is strongly associated with the probability of responding (Z = 3.86, p = 0.0001). The estimated relationship is specified by the equation

$$Pr(Y = 1 | d) = \frac{e^{-1.92 + 2.78d}}{1 + e^{-1.92 + 2.78d}},$$

and Figure 11.1 is actually a plot of this estimated dependence of $Pr(Y = 1 | d)$ on dose.

In many dose-response problems, the estimation of the median effective dose, which is denoted by ED_{50}, is of particular interest. The ED_{50} value is the actual dose required to induce the designated response in 50% of the population. Since $Pr(Y = 1 | d = ED_{50}) = Pr(Y = 0 | d = ED_{50}) = 0.5$, it follows that

$$\log \left\{ \frac{Pr(Y = 1 | d = ED_{50})}{Pr(Y = 0 | d = ED_{50})} \right\} = \log(0.5/0.5)$$

$$= 0 = a + b(ED_{50});$$

therefore $ED_{50} = -a/b$ and its estimated value is $\hat{ED}_{50} = -\hat{a}/\hat{b}$. For the data analyzed in Table 11.9 the estimated ED_{50} is $-(-1.92)/2.78 = 0.69$, which corresponds to a concentration of $\exp(0.69) = 1.99$ mg/kg. The derivation of a 95% confidence interval for this concentration is somewhat complicated, since the ED_{50} estimate is itself a ratio of estimates. Readers are advised to consult a statistician if a confidence interval of this type is required. In this particular case, most approaches to the technical problem of deriving a confidence interval for ED_{50} would yield an interval which is approximately $(0.43, 0.95)$. The 95% confidence interval for the corresponding concentration is therefore $(e^{0.43}, e^{0.95}) = (1.54, 2.59)$. The derivation of estimates and confidence intervals for other doses or concentrations which are similarly defined is handled in a corresponding way.

To illustrate some special aspects of the use of logistic regression methods we now consider a combined analysis of the dose-response data for two of the patient groups described by *Duncan* et al. [1984]. The first set of patients (Group 1) consists of 94 children who did not receive premedication, whereas the second set (Group 2) consists of the 137 children premedicated orally with TDP and atropine. The regression model which was fitted to these data involves three covariates, X_1, X_2 and X_3. The binary variable X_1 takes the value 0 if a patient did not receive premedication and 1 if the patient received TDP and atropine. The variable X_2 corresponds to the logarithm of the concentration of thiopentone administered, i.e., the dosage d, while the covariate X_3 represents an interaction term which is formed by multiplying X_1 and X_2. Thus, X_3 is equal to the dosage, d, for patients in Group 2 and takes the value 0 for patients in Group 1. This means that the fitted model consists of two different forms, one for each group of patients. These two forms are

$$
\Pr(Y = 1 | d) = \begin{cases} \dfrac{\exp(a + b_2 d)}{1 + \exp(a + b_2 d)} & \text{for Group 1,} \\[3mm] \dfrac{\exp(a + b_1 + b_2 d + b_3 d)}{1 + \exp(a + b_1 + b_2 d + b_3 d)} & \text{for Group 2.} \end{cases} \tag{11.3}
$$

Notice that a and b_2 in the model for Group 1 are replaced in the model for Group 2 by $(a + b_1)$ and $(b_2 + b_3)$, respectively. The regression coefficients b_1 and b_3 reflect two kinds of differences between the patient groups. To understand these differences, let $p_1(d)$ and $p_2(d)$ be the probabilities of responding to dose level d of the anaesthetic in Groups 1 and 2, respectively. Then the odds ratio (OR) for Group 2 versus Group 1 is

Table 11.10. Maximum likelihood fit of a binary logistic regression model to data on 231 children anaesthetized with thiopentone

Coefficient	Estimate	Estimated standard error	z-statistic
a	-5.59	1.32	–
b_1	3.67	1.56	2.35 ($p = 0.02$)
b_2	3.33	0.79	4.22 ($p < 0.0001$)
b_3	-0.55	1.06	0.52 ($p = 0.60$)

A total of 137 children were premedicated with TDP and atropine; the remaining 94 did not receive premedication.

$$\frac{p_2(d)/\{1-p_2(d)\}}{p_1(d)/\{1-p_1(d)\}} = \frac{\exp(a + b_1 + b_2d + b_3d)}{\exp(a + b_2d)} = \exp(b_1 + b_3d).$$

If b_1 and b_3 are both zero, then this odds ratio is 1 and the probability of responding is identical in both groups. If $b_3 = 0$ then the odds ratio at all dose levels has the same value, namely $\exp(b_1)$. Thus, the dependence on dose is the same in both groups of patients and is described by the coefficient b_2. However, if $b_3 \neq 0$, then the dose dependence is different in the two groups, and therefore the odds ratio changes with dose by a factor $\exp(b_3d)$.

Table 11.10 presents the estimation of model (11.3). The regression coefficients for X_1 (Group 2) and X_2 (dose) are both significant, but the coefficient for X_3 is not significant. Thus, the dependence on dose of the probability of responding to thiopentone is the same in the two groups of patients. However, the actual probability of responding is higher for the group of patients who were premedicated with TDP and atropine. This difference between the two patient groups is reflected in the odds ratio, $\exp(b_1)$, which has an estimated value of $\exp(\hat{b}_1) = \exp(3.67) = 39.3$.

12 Proportional Hazards Regression

12.1. Introduction

In studies of chronic disease, perhaps the most frequent endpoint of interest is survival. In chapter 6, we introduced the Kaplan-Meier estimated survival curve and in chapter 7, the comparison of two survival curves via the log-rank test was described. In this chapter, we consider regression models for survival data. As with other regression models, the simultaneous influence of a number of explanatory variables can be investigated with these models. However, the models themselves have been designed to be particularly suited to survival data.

Throughout this section, we will refer to survival time as our endpoint of interest. As with chapter 6, however, the methodology applies to data arising as the time to a well-defined event. In cancer clinical trials, for example, the variable time to relapse or death is frequently used.

Two characteristics of survival data led to the development of regression models specific to this type of data. The first was the frequent occurrence of incomplete observation. If a number of patients are being followed to estimate the characteristics of a survival function, a fraction of these patients will very likely still be alive at the time of analysis. Therefore, we do not have complete survival information on these patients. Nevertheless, the knowledge that they have survived for a certain period of time should be incorporated into the analysis.

The second characteristic of survival data that led to the development of new statistical methods is the distribution of typical survival times. Classical statistical theory, such as multiple linear regression, is usually not appropriate for clinical data. In most studies, the distribution of survival times is unknown and the distributions tend to vary widely from one disease to another. Either the statistical models must incorporate a wide class of distributions that may be less readily applied than the normal distribution, or we must use methods that do not assume a specific distribution at all. Our discussion of proportional hazards regression concentrates on methodology that adopts the latter approach.

In chapters 6 and 7, we discussed the survival experience of 64 patients with Stages II, III or IV non-Hodgkin's lymphoma. A comparison was made between those whose disease presented with clinical symptoms (B symptoms) and those whose disease was discovered indirectly (A symptoms). A strong survival advantage was attributed to those patients with A symptoms.

A natural question to ask is whether this difference could arise because these two patient groups differed with respect to other important prognostic factors. For illustration, we will consider two such factors, stage of disease and the presence of a bulky abdominal mass.

12.2. A Statistical Model for the Death Rate

When analyzing survival time, it is convenient to think in terms of the death rate. More generally, a failure rate can be defined for investigating the time to any other type of 'failure'. The technical name for a failure rate is the hazard rate; historically, the death rate was called the force of mortality.

The death rate is defined, in mathematical terms, as the probability of dying at a specified time t when it is known that the individual did not die before t. This definition may seem somewhat artificial. However, it is a convenient, general way of representing the same type of information as that implied by the question 'What is the probability of surviving two years after therapy if a patient has already survived one year?'.

We will denote a death rate at time t by the function d(t). To develop a regression model, we need to incorporate information which is coded as covariates $X_1, X_2, ..., X_k$. As before, it is convenient to refer to the set of covariates as $\underline{X} = \{X_1, X_2, ..., X_k\}$. Thus, in the regression model we define, we want to describe the quantity $d(t; \underline{x})$, which is the death rate for an individual with observed values of the covariates $X_1 = x_1, X_2 = x_2, ..., X_k = x_k$, or $\underline{x} = \{x_1, x_2, ..., x_k\}$. A convenient regression model for $d(t; \underline{x})$ is specified by the equation

$$\log\{d(t; \underline{x})\} = \log\{d_0(t)\} + \sum_{i=i}^{k} b_i x_i. \qquad (12.1)$$

The death rate function, $d_0(t)$, in equation (12.1) represents the death rate at time t for an individual whose covariate values are all zero, i.e., $X_1 = 0, X_2 = 0, \ldots, X_k = 0$. It is not important that a patient having all values of the covariates equal to zero be realistic. Rather, $d_0(t)$ is simply a reference point, and serves the same function as the coefficient a in the expression $a + \Sigma\, b_i x_i$ which we used in previous regression models. The difference which $d_0(t)$ incorporates is that $d_0(t)$ changes as t varies, whereas the coefficient a was a single numerical constant. This model was introduced by *Cox* [1972] and is frequently referred to as the Cox regression model.

A survival curve is a graph of the function $Pr(T > t)$, the probability of survival beyond time t. For those who remember some calculus, we remark that

$$Pr(T > t) = \exp\left\{ - \int_0^t d(y)dy \right\}.$$

Otherwise, it suffices to say that by specifying the death rate, $d(t)$, we identify the function $Pr(T > t)$. Moreover, in terms of $Pr(T > t)$, it can be shown that the regression equation (12.1) is equivalent to

$$Pr(T > t; \underline{x}) = \{Pr_0\, (T > t)\}^{\exp\left\{ \sum_{i=1}^{k} b_i x_i \right\}}, \qquad (12.2)$$

where $Pr_0\, (T > t)$ is the survival curve for a patient whose covariate values are all zero.

Once again, the most important aspect of the regression model (12.1) concerns the regression coefficients. If b_i is zero, then the associated covariate is not related to survival, or does not contain information on survival, when adjustment is made for the other covariates included in the model.

The model is also valuable, however, because it easily accommodates the two specific characteristics of survival data which we mentioned in §12.1. When we estimate the coefficients, the b_i's, it is easy, and is in fact preferable, not to assume anything about the death rate function $d_0(t)$. Thus, we do not need to specify any particular form for the distribution of the survival times, and the model is applicable in a wide variety of settings. Secondly, it turns out that it is very easy to incorporate the information that an individual has survived beyond time t, but the exact survival time is unknown, into the estimation of the regression coefficients. The details of the actual calculations are beyond the scope of this book but, as before, the model estimation can be summarized as a table of estimated regression coefficients and their corresponding estimated standard errors.

12.3. The Lymphoma Example

Table 12.1 records the estimated regression coefficients and standard errors for a Cox regression analysis of survival time for the 64 lymphoma patients described in chapter 7. Three covariates, X_1, X_2 and X_3 were defined as follows:

$$X_1 = \begin{cases} 1 & \text{if the disease is Stage IV,} \\ 0 & \text{otherwise;} \end{cases}$$

$$X_2 = \begin{cases} 1 & \text{if the patient presents with B symptoms,} \\ 0 & \text{otherwise;} \end{cases}$$

$$X_3 = \begin{cases} 1 & \text{if a large abdominal mass (> 10 cm) is present,} \\ 0 & \text{otherwise.} \end{cases}$$

Coincidentally, these covariates are all binary, although this is not a formal requirement of the proportional hazards regression model.

From Table 12.1, we see that all three covariates are related to survival, even after adjustment for the other covariates. Thus, for example, we can say that the prognostic importance of B symptoms is not due to differences in stage and abdominal mass status among patients in the two symptom groups.

With a proportional hazards or Cox regression model and binary covariates, the results of an analysis can easily be described in terms of relative risk. For example, the death rate for Stage IV patients is $\exp(\hat{b}_1) = \exp(1.38) = 3.97$ times as large as that for Stage II or III patients. The relative risk associated with Stage IV disease is therefore 3.97. The relative risks for B symptoms and bulky disease are $\exp(1.10) = 3.00$ and $\exp(1.74) = 5.70$, respectively.

In this regression model, the relative risks need to be calculated relative to a baseline set of patient characteristics. For our model with three binary

Table 12.1. The results of a proportional hazards regression analysis of survival time based on 64 advanced stage non-Hodgkin's lymphoma patients

Covariate	Regression coefficient	Estimated standard error	z-statistic
Stage IV disease	1.38	0.55	2.51 (p = 0.012)
B symptoms	1.10	0.41	2.68 (p = 0.007)
Bulky disease	1.74	0.69	2.52 (p = 0.012)

covariates, it is convenient to take $X_1 = 0$, $X_2 = 0$ and $X_3 = 0$ as the baseline characteristics. Then the estimated relative risk for an individual with $X_1 = x_1$, $X_2 = x_2$ and $X_3 = x_3$ is

$$\exp(\hat{b}_1 x_1 + \hat{b}_2 x_2 + \hat{b}_3 x_3). \tag{12.3}$$

For example, the relative risk for a Stage IV patient with B symptoms and bulky disease is $\exp(1.38 + 1.10 + 1.74) = 68.0$ compared to a Stage II or III patient with A symptoms and no abdominal mass. Estimated relative risks for such extreme comparisons should be interpreted with some skepticism, since the associated standard errors are frequently very large. It is also possible to examine whether the model specified in equation (12.3), which sums the three regression coefficients, is, in fact, reasonable. To do this, we would code additional covariates which represent patients having two or three of the characteristics of interest. If these extra covariates have non-zero regression coefficients, then they should be included in a revised model, and their inclusion will alter the additive relationship in equation (12.3).

For example, if we code a covariate X_4 as

$$X_4 = \begin{cases} 1 & \text{if a patient has B symptoms and Stage IV disease} \\ 0 & \text{otherwise,} \end{cases}$$

then the estimated regression model including X_1, X_2, X_3 and X_4 has regression coefficients $\hat{b}_1 = 2.17$, $\hat{b}_2 = 1.98$, $\hat{b}_3 = 1.66$ and $\hat{b}_4 = -1.07$. The coefficient for X_4 has an associated p-value of 0.36. From this model, the estimated relative risk for a Stage IV patient with B symptoms and bulky disease is $\exp(2.17 + 1.98 + 1.66 - 1.07) = 114.4$. This estimate is presented solely for the purposes of illustration, since the p-value of 0.36, which is associated with a test of the hypothesis $b_4 = 0$, does not support the use of a model incorporating X_4. In fact, with a small data set, a model involving a covariate which represents several factors combined usually would not be considered.

The recognition that regression coefficients are only estimates is more important than the particular estimates of relative risk which can be calculated. As we indicated in chapter 8, we can calculate confidence intervals for regression coefficients. The 95% confidence interval for b_i is defined to be

$$\hat{b}_i \pm 1.96 \{\text{est. standard error } (\hat{b}_i)\}.$$

If we represent this interval by (b_{iL}, b_{iH}), then, for a Cox regression model, we can also obtain a 95% confidence interval for the relative risk, $\exp(b_i)$, namely

$$(\exp(b_{iL}), \exp(b_{iH})).$$

Table 12.2. Estimates of the 95% confidence intervals for regression coefficients and relative risks corresponding to the model analyzed in Table 12.1

Covariate	Regression coefficient	95% Confidence interval	Relative risk	95% Confidence interval
Stage IV disease	1.38	(0.30, 2.46)	3.97	(1.35, 11.68)
B symptoms	1.10	(0.30, 1.90)	3.00	(1.35, 6.71)
Bulky disease	1.74	(0.39, 3.09)	5.70	(1.47, 22.03)

Table 12.2 presents estimated regression coefficients, relative risks and confidence intervals for the lymphoma example. Since there are only 64 patients, the confidence intervals are very wide; therefore, little importance should be attached to any of the estimates. Any discussion of estimation based on regression models should clearly indicate the potential error in the estimates. Remember, also, that a 'significant' regression coefficient ($p < 0.05$) merely means that a 95% confidence interval for the regression coefficient excludes the value zero.

It is not possible to discuss, in one brief chapter, all the intricacies of a proportional hazards regression model. We would suggest that a statistician be involved if this model is used extensively in the analysis of any data set. However, there is one remaining feature of the model which merits some discussion.

Any regression model is based on a particular, assumed relationship between the dependent variable and the explanatory covariates. It is important to examine the validity of this assumed relationship. It need not have a biological basis, but it must be a reasonable, empirical description of the observed data. Most regression models allow the model assumption to be examined.

The assumption of the Cox regression model which is discussed most often is that of proportional hazards. Equation (12.1) implies that

$$d(t; \underline{x}) = \{d_0(t)\} \times \exp\left\{\sum_{i=1}^{k} b_i x_i\right\},$$

which specifies that the death rate for an individual with covariate values $\underline{x}$ is a constant multiple, $\exp\{\sum b_i x_i\}$, of the baseline death rate *at all times*. Thus, although the death rate $d_0(t)$ can change with time, the ratio of the death rates, $d(t; \underline{x})/d_0(t)$, is always equal to $\exp\{\sum b_i x_i\}$.

Table 12.3. The results of a proportional hazards regression analysis of survival time, stratified by stage of disease; the analysis is based on 64 advanced stage non-Hodgkin's lymphoma patients

Covariate	Regression coefficient	Estimated standard error	z-statistic
B symptoms	1.11	0.41	2.71 (p = 0.007)
Bulky disease	1.80	0.69	2.61 (p = 0.010)

The proportional hazards regression model is frequently criticized for this assumption but, in fact, it is very easy to generalize the model to accommodate a time-dependent hazard or death rate ratio. In the following discussion, we indicate a simple approach which is useful in many situations.

Let us suppose that we do not want to assume that the death rate for Stage IV patients is a constant multiple of that for Stage II or III patients, and we do not have any information concerning the actual nature of the relationship. In this case, two regression equations can be defined as follows:

$$\log\{d_1(t; x_2, x_3)\} = \log\{d_{01}(t)\} + b_2 x_2 + b_3 x_3$$

and

$$\log\{d_2(t; x_2, x_3)\} = \log\{d_{02}(t)\} + b_2 x_2 + b_3 x_3,$$

where $d_1(t; x_2, x_3)$ is the death rate for Stage II or III patients and $d_2(t; x_2, x_3)$ is the death rate for Stage IV patients. Notice that the regression coefficients for B symptoms and bulky disease are assumed to be the same in the two regression equations. This is called a stratified version of Cox's regression model, and it is an extremely useful generalization of the basic proportional hazards regression model.

Table 12.3 presents estimates and standard errors of b_2 and b_3 based on this stratified model. In Table 12.1, the test that b_2 or b_3 could be equal to zero was adjusted for any possible confounding effects of disease stage by the inclusion of the covariate X_1 in the regression model. In Table 12.3, the corresponding tests are adjusted because the model is stratified by disease stage. This latter adjustment is more general, in that it does not assume there is any specific relationship between $d_1(t; x_2, x_3)$ and $d_2(t; x_2, x_3)$, whereas, in Table 12.1, the assumption has been made that

$$d_2(t; x_2, x_3) = d_1(t; x_2, x_3) \exp(b_1).$$

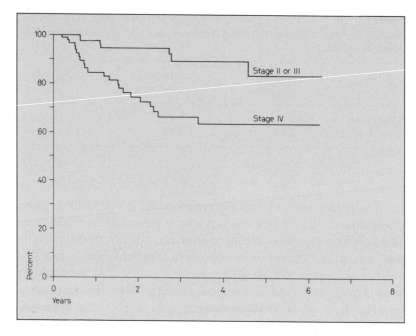

Fig. 12.1. The estimated survival curves for non-Hodgkin's lymphoma patients with A symptoms and no bulky disease, stratified by disease stage.

In this example, the conclusions with respect to b_2 and b_3 are hardly altered by the use of the stratified model. This will not always be the case, of course. When a stratified model is used, it is possible to estimate the baseline functions $d_{01}(t)$ and $d_{02}(t)$. This means, in our particular example, that we can estimate survival curves for patients with A symptoms and no bulky disease, subdivided by disease stage (II or III versus IV). Figure 12.1 presents these estimates graphically. The method of estimation will not be discussed here. It is a generalization of the techniques which we discussed in chapter 6. If we then multiply the estimates of $d_{01}(t)$ and $d_{02}(t)$ by $\exp\{\hat{b}_2 x_2 + \hat{b}_3 x_3\}$, we can generate the corresponding survival curves for patients with covariate values $X_2 = x_2$ and $X_3 = x_3$. For example, Figure 12.2 presents the curves for patients with B symptoms and bulky disease.

If we wish to examine whether a proportional hazard assumption is reasonable for representing the effect of disease stage (II or III versus IV), then Figure 12.1 can be replotted on a log(–log) scale. This is done in Figure 12.3. If the two estimated survival curves are parallel, then the ratio of the

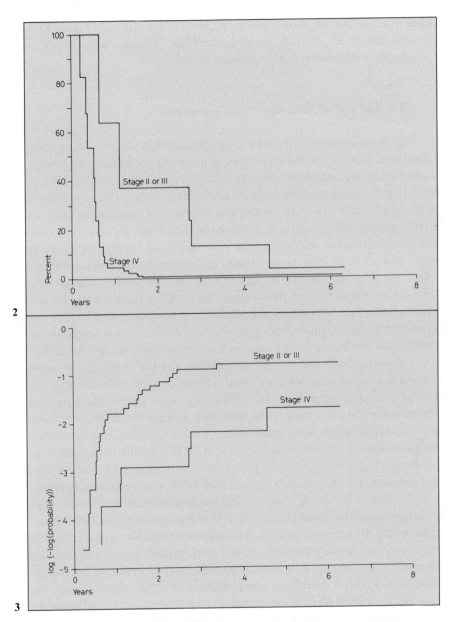

Fig. 12.2. The estimated survival curves for non-Hodgkin's lymphoma patients with B symptoms and bulky disease, stratified by disease stage.

Fig. 12.3. The estimated survival curves shown in Figure 12.1 plotted on a log(–log) scale.

death rates for the two patient groups is constant over time. In Figure 12.3, the two curves are roughly parallel; therefore, it seems appropriate to include X_1 in an unstratified regression model.

12.4. The Use of Time-Dependent Covariates

The lymphoma example which was discussed in the previous section introduces most of the basic features of proportional hazards regression, with one notable exception. All the explanatory variables in the regression model for the death rate represent patient characteristics which are defined at the start of the follow-up period, and this initial classification does not change throughout the analysis. Covariates of this type are said to be fixed with respect to time, and commonly arise in clinical studies. However, in some situations it may be desirable, and appropriate, to examine the influence on a hazard rate of patient characteristics which change over time. In the remainder of this section, we describe such a situation and illustrate the ease with which time-dependent covariates can be incorporated into proportional hazards regression. In our view, it is a very attractive feature of this regression approach to the analysis of survival data.

Following bone marrow transplantation for the treatment of acute leukemia, an important outcome event is the recurrence of the disease. The rate of leukemic relapse can be modelled using a proportional hazards regression of the time from transplantation to leukemic relapse. Another serious complication which may arise in the immediate post-transplant period is acute graft-versus-host disease (GVHD), which is thought to be an immunologic reaction of the new marrow graft against the patient. The interrelationship of these two adverse outcomes is of particular interest.

Prentice et al. [1978] examine this interrelationship by incorporating information on the occurrence of GVHD in a proportional hazards regression model for leukemic relapse following bone marrow transplantation. However, the development of GVHD in a patient is not a predictable phenomenon. Therefore, it would be quite inappropriate to model the effect of GVHD on the relapse rate by using a covariate which ignores this fact, i.e., by using a fixed covariate which classifies an individual as having GVHD throughout the post-transplant period. The simplest possible way to incorporate this temporal dependence would involve the use of a binary covariate which is equal to zero at times prior to a diagnosis of GVHD, but takes the value one at all times thereafter. If more comprehensive data are

Table 12.4. The results of a proportional hazards regression analysis of leukemia relapse data based on 135 patients treated for acute leukemia by means of bone marrow transplantation

Covariate	Regression coefficient	Estimated standard error	z-statistic
GVHD	−0.76	0.37	2.05 (p = 0.04)
Transplant type	0.05	0.34	0.15 (p = 0.88)
Age	0.13	0.10	1.30 (p = 0.19)

Adapted from *Prentice* et al. [1978] with permission from the Biometric Society.

available, perhaps indicating the severity of GVHD, this information could also be incorporated into the regression model through the use of suitably defined time-dependent covariates.

In §12.2, we used the notation, d(t), to represent the dependence of a death rate on time. Here we will denote a relapse rate by r(t) and, in a similar fashion, use X(t) to show the dependence of a covariate on time. Let $\underline{X}(t) = \{X_1(t), \ldots, X_k(t)\}$ represent the set of covariates in the regression model. Then for an individual with observed values of the covariates $\underline{x}(t) = \{x_1(t), \ldots, x_k(t)\}$, a regression equation for the leukemic relapse rate, which parallels equation (12.1), is

$$\log\{r(t;\underline{x}(t))\} = \log\{r_0(t)\} + \sum_{i=1}^{k} b_i x_i(t).$$

The addition of time-dependent covariates to the model is a very natural extension of equation (12.1), which already included a dependence on time. Although this refinement of the proportional hazards model appears to be simply a change in notation, it represents a major advance in biostatistical technique. There are many subtleties associated with its use and interpretation which we are not able to discuss adequately in these few pages. Readers are strongly urged to consult a statistician from the very beginning of any proposed study that may eventually involve the use of time-dependent covariates in a regression model.

Table 12.4, which is taken from *Prentice* et al. [1978], presents the results of an analysis of data on leukemic relapse in 135 patients. Since the sample includes 31 syngeneic (identical twin) bone marrow transplants with no risk of GVHD, the regression model includes a binary covariate indicating the type of transplant (0 = syngeneic, 1 = allogeneic) and a continuous covariate representing patient age (years/10). As the results of this analysis indicate, neither of these covariates is significantly associated with leukemic relapse. However, their inclusion in the model adjusts the estimation of the GVHD effect for the influence of transplant type and patient age. Even after adjusting for the effect of these variables, the regression coefficient for GVHD is significant at the 0.05 level. The rate of leukemic relapse for patients who develop GVHD is estimated to be $\exp(-0.76) = 0.47$ times the relapse rate for patients who do not have GVHD at the same time post-transplant. The corresponding 95% confidence interval for this relative risk is $(e^{-1.46}, e^{-0.03}) = (0.23, 0.97)$.

The results of this analysis suggest that the occurrence of GVHD is protective with respect to leukemic relapse. This may indicate that GVHD serves to eradicate residual or new leukemic cells. The clinical implications of this finding are, of course, subtle and will not be discussed here. However, it may be that although severe GVHD is clearly undesirable, a limited graft-versus-host reaction could help to control leukemic relapse.

In the last three chapters, we have presented a brief introduction to the concept of regression models. Without a much longer exposition of these topics, we can only hope that our discussion has helped readers to acquire some understanding of these important techniques, and has rendered their use in research papers somewhat less mysterious.

13 Data Analysis

13.1. Introduction

In the preceding chapters, we have discussed a number of statistical techniques which are used in the analysis of medical data. It has generally been assumed that a well-defined set of data is available, to which a specific procedure is to be applied. In this chapter, we adopt a broader perspective in order to address some general aspects of data analysis.

There is a necessary formalism to most statistical calculations which is often not consistent with their application. While the formal properties of statistical tests do indicate their general characteristics, their specific application to a particular problem can require adaptation and compromise. Data analysis, perhaps, is as much an art as it is a science.

Experience is the only good introduction to data analysis. Our aim, in this chapter, is to highlight a few principles with which the reader should be familiar. These should promote a more informed reading of the medical literature, and lead to a deeper understanding of the potential role of statistics in personal research activity. Where possible, we will use examples for illustration although, since they are chosen for this purpose, these examples may be simpler than many genuine research problems. Also, any analysis which we present should not be considered definitive, since alternative approaches may very well be possible.

13.2. Quality Data

'Garbage in, garbage out' is an apt description of the application of statistics to poor data. Thus, although it may be obvious, it is worth stressing the importance of high-quality data.

If information is collected on a number of individuals, then it is critical that the nature of the information be identical for all individuals. Any classification of patients must follow well-defined rules which are uniformly applied. For example, if a number of pathologists are classifying tumors, there should be a mechanism to check that the classification is consistent from one pathologist to another. This might involve a re-review of all slides by a single pathologist, or selected cases could be used as consistency checks.

Of course, it is possible that data may be missing for some individuals. Provided that a consistent effort has been applied to collect data, allowance for the missing data can frequently be made in a statistical analysis. Even then, however, if there are observable differences in a response variable between individuals with and individuals without particular information, any conclusions based only on those individuals with available data may be suspect.

Two major types of data collection can be identified; we shall call the two approaches retrospective and prospective. Retrospective data collection refers to data which were recorded at some previous time and subsequently are selected to be used for research purposes. The quality of retrospective data is often out of the control of the investigator. Good detective work may provide the best information available, but what is available may vary widely from individual to individual. For retrospective data, classification frequently must be based on the greatest amount of information which is available on all patients. For example, it has been shown that prior blood transfusions are associated with a poorer prognosis for aplastic anemia patients undergoing bone marrow transplantation. Patient records from the time prior to their arrival at the transplant center contained varying details on transfusion histories. As a result, early studies were necessarily limited to a simple binary classification as to whether any blood transfusions had been given or not, even though, for some patients, the number of units of blood received could be identified.

Prospective data collection generally occurs in a well-designed study. In such a situation, specified information is identified to be of interest, and this information is collected as it becomes available. The problem which arises in this type of study is one of ensuring that the information is, in fact, recorded at all, and is recorded accurately. In large collaborative studies this is a major concern, and can require considerable staff over and above the necessary medical care personnel.

Some additional aspects of data collection will be mentioned in chapter 14, which discusses the design of medical studies. In the rest of this chapter, only analyses of available data will be considered.

Table 13.1. Some information collected by questionnaires from 180 pregnant women

---

1 Patient number
2 Back pain severity
  (0) 'nil'
  (1) 'nothing worth troubling about'
  (2) 'troublesome, but not severe'
  (3) 'severe'
3 Age of patient (years)
5 Height of patient (meters)
6 Weight of patient at start of pregnancy (kg)
7 Weight of patient at end of pregnancy (kg)
8 Weight of baby (kg)
9 Number of children by previous pregnancies
10 Does the patient have a history of backache with previous pregnancy?
  (1) 'not applicable'
  (2) 'no'
  (3) 'yes, mild'
  (4) 'yes, severe'
13 Does walking aggravate back pain? (no/yes)

13.3. Initial or Exploratory Analysis

Before any formal statistical analysis can begin, the nature of the available data and the questions of interest need to be considered. In designed studies with careful data collection, this phase of analysis is simplified. It is always wise, however, to confirm that data are what they should be, especially if subsequent analyses involve computer manipulation of the data.

Table 13.1 presents a subset of some information obtained by questionnaires from 180 pregnant women [*Mantle* et al., 1977]. The data were collected to study back pain in pregnancy and, more particularly, to relate the severity of back pain to other items of information. The results of the questionnaires were kindly made available by Dr. *Mantle* to a workshop on data analysis sponsored by the Royal Statistical Society.

In this example, as in many medical studies, there is a clearly defined response variable which is to be related to other explanatory variables. If the response variable is not obvious, then it is important to consider whether such a distinction among the variables can be made, because it does influence the focus of the analysis.

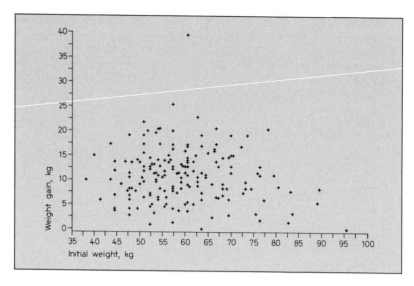

Fig. 13.1. A scatterplot of weight gain during pregnancy versus weight at the start of pregnancy for 180 women.

The initial phase of an analysis consists of simple tabulations or graphical presentations of the available data. For example, Figure 13.1 is a scatterplot of weight gain in pregnancy versus weight at the start of pregnancy. The most obvious feature of this plot is that one woman has a recorded weight gain of almost 40 kg, about twice that of the woman with the next largest weight gain. This is somewhat suspicious and should be checked. Such extreme values can seriously influence estimation procedures. Also, two women are identified as having a zero weight gain; the weights at the start and end of pregnancy recorded on their questionnaires were identical. Although this is not impossible, such data should also be checked. Since we cannot verify the available data, these three individuals will be omitted from subsequent analyses.

Table 13.2 is a table of the responses to a question about a history of backache in previous pregnancies and the number of children by previous pregnancies. This highlights another problem with the quality of the available data. Although the response to the question concerning a history of backache in previous pregnancies was supposed to be coded 1, 2, 3 or 4, 26 women coded the value 0. Also, two women with no children by prior pregnancies

Table 13.2. The responses to question 10 cross-tabulated by the responses to question 9 (see Table 13.1)

Number of children by previous pregnancies	History of backache with previous pregnancies			
	0	1 ≡ not applicable	2 ≡ no	3/4 ≡ mild/severe
0	20	79	1	1
≥ 1	6	4	32	37

Table 13.3. The revised responses to question 10 cross-tabulated by the responses to question 9 (see Tables 13.1, 13.2)

Number of children by previous pregnancies	History of backache with previous pregnancies			
	not applicable	no	mild	severe
0	101	0	0	0
1	0	28	19	5
2	0	6	3	3
3	0	3	4	0
4	0	3	0	0
5	0	1	2	0
6	0	0	0	1
7	0	1	0	0

have recorded codes concerning back pain, and four women with previous pregnancies have recorded responses labelled not applicable. If possible, these responses should also be checked, but here we are forced to make the 'reasonable' assumption that the not applicable and zero codes for women with previous pregnancies correspond to no previous backache (coded 2), and we recode the responses for all women with no previous pregnancies as 1 (not applicable). To shorten the discussion, we shall ignore the possibility of miscarriage, etc.

One aim of these preliminary tabulations, then, is to clean up the data set. This can be a time-consuming operation in a large data set, where the consistency of many variables needs to be checked. However, inconsistencies must be resolved, and this sort of activity is an important component of data analysis.

Table 13.3 is an expanded version of Table 13.2 after the miscoded responses have been revised. This table indicates that the majority of the women have had no children, or at most one child, by a previous pregnancy. For the few women with more than one child by previous pregnancies, the degree of back pain does not depend strongly on the number of pregnancies. Therefore, without performing any formal statistical tests, we might conclude that there is little to be gained from a detailed study of the number of children by previous pregnancies. Initially, formal analysis procedures may therefore be restricted to considering the simple binary classification of parous and nulliparous women.

We will not discuss any additional exploratory investigation of these data. Nevertheless, exploratory analysis is important, and we hope some appreciation for this aspect of data analysis has been conveyed.

13.4. Primary Analysis

In many medical studies, there are clearly defined questions of primary interest. In a clinical trial, for example, the treatment comparison is the main purpose of the trial; any additional information is of secondary importance, or has been collected to aid in making a valid treatment comparison. We will assume that, in the back pain example we have been discussing, the primary purpose was an initial study of the influence on backache of unalterable factors such as age and previous pregnancies. This suggests that adjustment may be required for other factors such as weight gain during pregnancy. Regression models are frequently a useful method of analysis in such a situation.

In this study, the response variable, back pain, is of a type we have not previously discussed in the context of regression models. It is discrete, with four categories, and is naturally ordered. Regression models for such data do exist, extending, in principle, the ideas of logistic regression. However, the primary purpose of the analysis may not require the use of such a specialized technique. More important yet, we should consider whether the data warrant a highly sophisticated treatment. Reaction to pain is likely to be very variable among individuals. Because of this, it may not be sensible to use a method of analysis which places importance on the distinction between the back pain categories 'nil' and 'nothing worth troubling about'. Similarly, the distinction between the upper two levels, 'troublesome' and 'severe', may not represent reliable data. For the primary purpose of the study, therefore, let us divide

Table 13.4. Current back pain severity versus a history of backache with previous pregnancies

History of backache with previous pregnancies	Current back pain severity				Total
	none	little	troublesome	severe	
Not applicable	8	56	28	9	101
None	5	14	14	9	42
Mild	0	7	13	8	28
Severe	0	3	5	1	9
Total	13	80	60	27	180

Table 13.5. The results of a logistic regression analysis relating back pain in pregnancy to a history of backache in previous pregnancies and age

Covariate		Coefficient	Standard error	z-statistic	Significance level (p-value)
a		−0.61	0.23	−	−
Age < 20 years		0.13	0.47	0.28	0.78
Age > 30 years		0.14	0.40	0.35	0.73
History of backache in previous pregnancies	none	0.64	0.39	1.64	0.10
	mild	1.64	0.50	3.28	0.001
	severe	1.23	0.75	1.64	0.10

Table 13.6. The logistic regression coefficients and estimated standard errors for weight gain variables added to the logistic model specified in Table 13.5

Covariate	Added singly		Added jointly	
	coefficient	standard error	coefficient	standard error
Actual weight gain	0.07	0.03	−0.58	0.34
Fractional weight gain	3.91	1.83	−5.18	6.17
Actual weight gain/height	0.13	0.05	1.20	0.62

the back pain variable into two categories which represent the upper and lower two levels of response, assuming that this distinction will be realistic and meet the needs of the analysis. Logistic regression then becomes a natural choice for the method of analysis.

There are a variety of approaches to the use of logistic regression and the identification of important covariates which should be included in any model. Table 13.4 suggests that there is a relationship between a history of back pain in pregnancy and pain in the pregnancy under study. This variable would likely be included in a model. Notice that this information will require three covariates in the logistic model. The baseline category consists of nulliparous women. The three binary covariates are used to compare women in the three pain categories of none, mild and severe to this baseline category. Age of the patient is also a covariate of interest, and would be considered for inclusion in the model.

Table 13.5 presents the results of a logistic regression analysis which incorporates these two variables. The model indicates that the historical covariates are associated with current pain. Notice that the variable comparing parous women with no history of backache to nulliparous women is the least significant of the three historical comparison covariates and has a considerably smaller coefficient than the other two historical variables. If the coefficients for these three variables were comparable, we might suggest using a single variable comparing parous and nulliparous women. Since the coefficients for the variables coding mild and severe pain in previous pregnancies are comparable, it suggests that the important predictive distinctions would be between women who are nulliparous, parous with no history and parous with some history of backache in previous pregnancies.

The coefficients for age are not significant in Table 13.5, indicating that age is not related to back pain in pregnancy after adjustment for the historical backache information. In fact, age is not important, even if examined alone.

Conventional wisdom would suggest that weight gain in pregnancy will influence back pain. As is frequently the case, however, there are a variety of ways that weight gain could be introduced into the logistic regression model. Consider the three possibilities of actual weight gain, weight gain as a fraction of initial weight and actual weight gain divided by height. The last two variables attempt to take into account the influence of physical characteristics of a woman in carrying a child.

Table 13.6 records the logistic regression coefficients for each of these variables when added to the model specified in Table 13.5. Also recorded are the coefficients when all three variables are added simultaneously. The most significant variable appears to be actual weight gain divided by height.

On the basis of these calculations, it would be customary to include actual weight gain/height and the historical pain variables in the logistic regression analysis presented in Table 13.7. In a paper, Table 13.7 might appear as a summary of the logistic regression analysis. The means of arriving at this model has been entirely suppressed, but this should influence our interpretation of the stated p-values.

The variables relating to historical pain are straightforward, and the associated p-values are indicative of their relationship to back pain. However, the variable actual weight gain/height was chosen from a pool of other possible covariates precisely because it had a low p-value. This is one version of something called the 'multiple comparisons problem'. This issue frequently arises when regression techniques are used, and the reader should be aware of it. Non-technically, the multiple comparisons problem can be described as statistical testing of effects suggested by the data. In any data set there will be peculiarities, and if one searches long enough, they can be found.

As a simple illustration of this problem, consider the averages of some variable in four groups of individuals. If the highest average is compared with the lowest average using a simple t-test, then the p-value will be artificially low because there must be a highest value and a lowest value, and even if there are no real differences between the groups, the expected difference between the observed highest and lowest values must be positive. Perhaps this illustration is a statistical counterpart of the aphorism 'There is nothing you can't prove if your outlook is only sufficiently limited'.

In our analysis of the back pain data, the inclusion of a weight gain variable is important principally because it establishes an independent effect for the historical information on back pain in previous pregnancies. From this perspective, the choice between roughly comparable variables is not critical. No great importance should be attached to the form of the variable unless it is clearly more useful for predictive purposes than other choices in a variety of studies.

These general reservations concerning the uncritical interpretation of p-values in the context of multiple comparisons should be kept in mind, although it is difficult to formalize them. In §13.6, some formal consideration will be given to the same problem in a different context.

Although we have not presented all the details here, the logistic regression analysis will allow us to answer the primary questions of the back pain

Table 13.7. A logistic regression analysis of the 'final' model for back pain in pregnancy

Covariate		Coefficient	Standard error	z-statistic	Significance level (p-value)
a		−1.49	0.44	–	–
History of backache in previous pregnancies	none	0.73	0.39	1.87	0.06
	mild	1.76	0.49	3.59	<0.001
	severe	1.41	0.75	1.88	0.06
Actual weight gain/height		0.13	0.05	2.60	0.01

study. The experience of previous pregnancies is important in predicting back pain in pregnancy, while age is not important. This conclusion remains valid, even after adjustment for other variables which may also influence back pain.

13.5. Secondary Analyses

To answer the primary questions of a study, a degree of conservatism is usually wise. Often, the analyses undertaken should have been specified before the data were collected. The assumptions of any statistical model used should be consistent with the observed data, or seen as convenient simplifications which help to summarize the data without affecting the major conclusions.

After this phase of the analysis has been completed, additional data analysis is often undertaken. The distinction between primary and secondary analyses is not well-defined and frequently is not made at all. The reason we emphasize it here is to convey the notion that, in some settings, it is wise to downplay the importance of formal statistical tests.

For example, consider the back pain study which we discussed in §§13.3, 13.4. Factors which influence whether a woman with pain will call it severe or not may be of interest. Although this judgement may be quite subjective and variable, it is appropriate to look at data of this type.

For the 84 women in the back pain study who reported troublesome or severe pain, Table 13.8 presents a logistic regression analysis with covariates

Table 13.8. The results of a logistic regression analysis of severe versus troublesome pain

Covariate	Coefficient	Standard error	z-statistic	Significance level (p-value)
a	−1.51	0.39	–	–
Age < 20 years	−0.22	0.82	0.27	0.79
Age > 30 years	1.39	0.55	2.53	0.01
Walking aggravates pain	1.40	0.62	2.26	0.02

which distinguish between these two categories. The covariates which discriminate between no pain and some pain, namely a history of backache and weight gain, do not discriminate between the upper two pain categories. Rather, the important covariates are age and an indication of whether walking aggravates pain. The effect of walking is only relevant to this logistic model since the patient must experience pain in order to aggravate it. Medically, one might speculate that this variable is a proxy for walking with bad posture, and plan to address this question in a later study. The fact that age plays an apparent role in the logistic model described in Table 13.8, but not in the primary model, is somewhat surprising. Unless there is some reason to expect such a discrepancy, it would be wise not to stress the importance of an age effect until it could be confirmed in a subsequent study.

The general attitude of reservation which is expressed in the preceding paragraph is appropriate because if one continues to look at subsets of the data, then it is likely that something interesting will be found. As a hypothesis-generating activity, that is, to suggest future research questions, secondary analysis is valuable. However, the nature of this activity does undermine the probabilistic ideas of formal significance tests; therefore, the interpretation of secondary analyses should be treated with some caution.

When secondary analyses identify quite marked effects or relationships, then there is no reason they should not appear in published research. Other researchers are then able to consider the possibility of observing similar findings in related situations. However, the nature of the analysis which led to the findings should be made clear. Finally, in reading published papers, it is wise to consider whether the findings which are reported suggest that some discounting of reported significance levels would be prudent.

Table 13.9. Data concerning the presence of the HLA allele B8 in a diabetic and a control population

	B8 present	B8 absent
Diabetics	30	47
Controls	28	113

13.6. A Formal Discussion of Multiple Comparisons

In §13.4, we introduced the problem of multiple comparisons. Our discussion of this issue was necessarily general because the problem is often difficult to formalize. In some situations, however, specific allowance can be made for multiple comparisons.

Consider a sample of 77 diabetics and 141 normal individuals for whom HLA typing is available. More specifically, we will assume that, for each individual, the presence of alleles B7, B8, B12, and B15 at the B-locus of the human leukocyte antigen system on chromosome 6 can be detected.

Table 13.9 records presence or absence data for allele B8 in the two populations. A χ^2 test of independence leads to an observed value for the test statistic of 8.35 and a p-value of 0.004. Such tables frequently appear in the medical literature.

What has been suppressed in this presentation of the data is the fact that B8 is one of four alleles that could have been detected, and a similar 2×2 table for each allele could be produced. Table 13.9 presents the 2×2 table which leads to the most significant p-value. Once again, we have a situation where a significance test has been chosen on the basis of observed data.

If the number of comparisons which were undertaken can be counted, then a theorem in theoretical statistics due to Bonferroni suggests that the p-value for each comparison should be multiplied by the total number of comparisons undertaken. Hence, an adjusted p-value for Table 13.9 would be $4(0.004) = 0.016$.

The appropriate application of the Bonferroni adjustment is not always clear, although it is a useful rule to keep in mind. When the results of such an adjustment are to be used to justify important conclusions, it would be prudent to seek statistical advice.

Table 13.10. Cross-tabulations of current back pain in pregnancy versus backache in previous pregnancies: **(a)** full table; **(b)** collapsed table

a Full table

Current back pain	Backache in previous pregnancies				Total
	not applicable	none	mild	severe	
None or mild	64 (52.18)[1]	19 (21.70)	7 (14.47)	3 (4.65)	93
Moderate or severe	37 (48.82)	23 (20.30)	21 (13.53)	6 (4.35)	87
Total	101	42	28	9	180

b Collapsed table

Current back pain	Backache in previous pregnancies			Total
	not applicable	none	mild or severe	
None or mild	64 (52.18)[1]	19 (21.70)	10 (19.12)	93
Moderate or severe	37 (48.82)	23 (20.30)	27 (17.88)	87
Total	101	42	37	180

[1] The values in parentheses are expected numbers if the row and column classifications are independent.

Another useful approach when multiple comparisons are a problem is known as the global test. Consider, for example, the relationship between previous backache and current back pain in pregnant women. Ignoring the effect of weight gain, Table 13.10a cross-tabulates backache in previous pregnancies by the two categories of current pain used in the logistic analyses which we discussed in §13.4.

One test of the hypothesis that the historical backache classification is independent of the current pain category is the χ^2 test for rectangular contingency tables discussed in §4.3. For this test, the observed value of the test statistic is 15.44 on $1 \times 3 = 3$ degrees of freedom. The 0.01 and 0.001 critical

Table 13.11. The results of a logistic regression analysis of diabetic status classified by HLA-B alleles

Covariate	Coefficient	Standard error	z-statistic	Significance level (p-value)
a	−0.72	0.27	–	–
B7	−0.65	0.40	1.63	0.10
B8	0.77	0.34	2.26	0.02
B12	−0.51	0.36	1.42	0.16
B15	0.71	0.37	1.92	0.05

values of a χ_3^2 distribution are 11.345 and 16.268, respectively, indicating that the p-value for this test of the hypothesis of independence lies between 0.01 and 0.001. There is, therefore, strong evidence of an association between backache in previous pregnancies and current back pain.

Although, in this example, there is strong evidence for a relationship between the two tabulated variables, it is often possible to increase the significance of a rectangular contingency table by choosing to pool certain categories. If the grouping is performed because it appears from the data that a smaller p-value can be obtained, then the observed p-value needs to be discounted. For example, if we group the mild and severe pain categories, as is done in Table 13.10b, then we can generate an observed value for the test statistic of 14.90 on two degrees of freedom, with a corresponding p-value which is less than 0.001.

Table 13.11 presents the results of a logistic regression analysis of diabetic status for the 218 individuals discussed at the beginning of this section. The model involves explanatory covariates which are binary, indicating the presence or absence of HLA-B alleles B7, B8, B12 and B15. For example, the covariate labelled B7 is equal to one if allele B7 is present on at least one of an individual's two chromosomes, and is equal to zero otherwise.

From Table 13.11, we see that allele B8 appears to have the strongest association with diabetic status. If we omit the other covariates, then in the resulting single covariate model involving variate B8 we would observe the same p-value of 0.004 as we saw previously in Table 13.9. It would be inappropriate to report this p-value, since the test was suggested by the less specific analysis of Table 13.11.

Even the results of Table 13.11 need to be interpreted carefully. The four covariates in Table 13.11 jointly classify the study subjects according to all available allelic information. However, each covariate also represents a simple classification of the individuals on the basis of a single allele. In the logistic regression analysis, one of the covariates must have the lowest p-value. Unless this particular classification was of prior interest, the observed p-value should be interpreted with caution.

With sets of classification variables such as the one we have described, a conservative approach to regression modelling involves a global test of the significance of the classification scheme. Formally, this is a test of the hypothesis that all the regression coefficients associated with the classification variables are zero. We have not previously discussed tests of this kind, but we can do so, briefly, at this point.

Corresponding to any estimated regression model, there is a number called the log-likelihood. If we have a regression model with a log-likelihood of L_1 and add k new covariates to the model, a new log-likelihood L_2 will result. If the null hypothesis that *all* the new covariates are unrelated to the dependent or response variable is true, the test statistic $T = 2(L_2 - L_1)$ is distributed, approximately, as a χ_k^2 random variable. A computer program is usually necessary to perform this global test, and a statistician should be consulted to carry out the detailed calculations and assist in interpreting the results of the test.

For the HLA data, the model presented in Table 13.11 would be compared with the simple one-parameter model which omits the four HLA-B classification variables. This leads to an observed value for T of 19.8. The 0.001 critical value for a χ_4^2 variate is 18.465; therefore, the p-value for the global test is less than 0.001. Since this global test of the HLA-B classification variables is significant, we can be more confident that the significant p-values for individual variables are not spurious.

It is impossible to present a comprehensive discussion of the complexities of data analysis, and the possible caveats which must be considered in presenting the results of a statistical analysis. However, we hope that this brief introduction will alert readers to some of the more important considerations.

14 The Design of Clinical Trials

14.1. Introduction

The main emphasis of this book is the analysis of medical data. The quality of data available for analysis clearly depends on the design for its collection, and a considerable number of general papers on the design of clinical trials have been written. In a medical trial, the investigators must balance considerations of ethics, simplicity and good statistical practice. It is often difficult, therefore, to give anything more than good, general advice about the characteristics of a well-designed study.

In this chapter, we shall briefly present a few of the issues which are frequently discussed. We also explore the role of randomized treatment assignment in clinical trials in somewhat greater detail. The use of randomized trials has been the subject of considerable debate, and we feel it deserves some discussion here. The technical matter of sample size in medical trials will be dealt with in the next chapter. Finally, we conclude the chapter with sections on factorial designs and repeated significance testing, two topics to which a brief introduction will be valuable.

14.2. General Considerations

Perhaps the primary requirement for a good clinical trial is that it should seek to answer an interesting question. The choice of treatments to be compared and the patients on whom they are to be compared largely determine the practical importance of discovering whether the treatments differ.

Strict entrance requirements which generate a very homogeneous patient population facilitate precise treatment comparisons with a small number of patients. However, the results of a larger study with a more heterogeneous population would probably be more convincing to a practising physician.

A trial with two highly divergent treatments is simple and is likely to produce a result more quickly than a trial with two similar treatments, or one involving more than two treatments. This observation is an important one since, for various reasons, it is often tempting to stop a trial before conclusive results have been obtained. On the other hand, sophisticated designs frequently allow more comprehensive inferences to be deduced. It is also important to ensure that the intended treatments are acceptable to the clinicians who must enroll their patients into the trial. Therefore, in selecting treatments, a balance must be struck among these various factors.

The design stage of a clinical trial should also specify data collection procedures. The information which will be collected concerning each patient at entry into the study should be identified. These baseline variables can be used in the analysis of the trial results to adjust for patient differences in the treatment arms. Therefore, information which is gathered at entry should be related to the chosen endpoints or to potential side effects of treatment; this latter aspect is sometimes overlooked. Since collecting data on a patient at the time of entry into a study is generally easier than attempting to recover relevant baseline information at a later time, it is advisable to record as much baseline data as is feasible.

Collecting data on only a few endpoints will make follow-up easier, and also reduces the chance of serious bias due to differential follow-up among patients. At the same time, as much information as possible should be recorded concerning each endpoint of the study. The time until a certain event is observed is more informative than a mere record of its occurrence. All patients who enter a trial should be followed, even if they abandon the treatment protocol, since exclusion of these patients can introduce bias. Similarly, the treatment groups which are compared in the primary analysis should be groups based on the treatments which were originally assigned, because this comparison reflects how the treatments will perform in practice. Of course, it may be of scientific interest to restrict a comparison to those patients receiving and tolerating treatment regimens, for example, but the more general comparison, based on assigned treatments, is usually more valuable in the long run. Note that, in order to avoid bias, treatment assignment should only occur after informed consent procedures.

Another point of frequent discussion concerns the stratification of treatment assignment by prognostic factors. The statistical methods which have been developed, such as regression models, reduce the need for precisely comparable treatment groups. It seems reasonable, however, to consider stratifying a trial on a few factors of known prognostic significance and to attempt partial balance on other factors via randomization. The effectiveness of the randomization in achieving this balance should be examined. *Peto* et al. [1976] argue in favor of no stratification, but it is more cautious, and perhaps more convincing, to balance on major prognostic factors rather than to rely solely on sophisticated statistical analyses to adjust for imbalances in the treatment arms. On the other hand, excessive stratification is complicated, unnecessary, and may even result in poor balance if only a few patients are entered in each stratum.

In the early design stage, the inferences which are to be drawn from the study should be identified. For example, suppose that a clinical trial of two adjuvant therapy regimens following surgery for breast cancer is being planned. The response variables which are of interest are remission duration and survival. The study protocol should specifically mention that remission duration and survival will be used to compare the two treatment regimens. In addition, the statistical procedure that will be used to analyze the results of the trial should be specified.

When the study has ended and the data are analyzed, it may be determined that the treatment A arm of the study had fewer metastases to the ovary than the treatment B arm, and this difference is statistically significant at the 5% level. Perhaps no other site of metastasis suggested there was a difference between the treatments, and the comparison of the two treatments on the basis of remission duration also indicated no difference. These results should not lead us to conclude that treatment A is better than B.

If ten sites of relapse were examined, then, because of the multiple comparisons problem which we discussed in chapter 13, it is not unlikely that one of the ten sites will, by accident, suggest there is a difference between treatments. If there was no reason, prior to the study, to suspect a treatment effect at a particular site of relapse, then the discovery of such an effect should be viewed with caution, especially if the designated principal comparison does not identify a treatment effect.

A major reason for specifying, in advance, the statistical procedure which will be used in the analysis is that it is possible to find perhaps ten different statistical tests which compare remission duration in two treatment groups. It might happen that one of these tests is just significant at the 5% level, while the rest suggest there is no significant difference. Such a 'search for significance' is entirely inappropriate; therefore, a reasonable test procedure should be specified before the study begins and used when the data are analyzed.

It may be that there is valid medical information in the unexpected results from a single relapse site, or that the statistical test indicating a treatment difference is particularly sensitive for the type of data produced by the study. If there is reason to suspect that this is the case, then the results should certainly be reported. How the results arose should also be reported, and it should be made clear that they need to be confirmed in other studies before being generally accepted. On the other hand, one can be much more confident about a result identified by a test which was specified prior to a detailed examination of the data.

14.3. Randomized versus Historical Controls

A randomized clinical trial is frequently used in clinical investigations. Nevertheless, there is considerable opposition to the use of such trials. One of the major concerns of those who oppose randomized trials is the ethical problem of allowing a random event to determine a patient's treatment.

We do not intend to summarize the array of arguments which have been advanced for and against randomized clinical trials. For those who wish to pursue further reading, a bibliography of papers may be found at the end of this chapter. Instead, we want to address the question of whether there are alternative designs which are as informative as a randomized trial. The issue is fundamental to all discussions of randomized trials.

We will assume that the purpose of a medical trial is to make a comparative statement about the efficacy of two or more treatments. Therefore, the accuracy of this statement is important. It has been argued that this particular assumption regarding a medical trial is inappropriate. *Freireich* [1983] has argued that a comparative trial which shows major differences between two treatments is a bad trial because half the patients have received inferior treatment. Although, in a sense, this is true, we feel that any wider perspective on clinical research will encompass a desire to know the true relative merits of different treatments.

If the purpose of a trial is to compare two treatments in a prospective fashion, then randomly assigning treatments to individuals as they enter the study should avoid many potential biasses which are present in other schemes for treatment assignment. In such a setting, some sort of randomization would usually not be objectionable.

Of more concern is the trial in which a new treatment is compared to an old treatment when there is information available about the efficacy of the old treatment through historical data. Patients who receive the old treatment are the controls against whom the patients who receive the new treatment are compared. Use of the historical data for comparisons with data from the new treatment will shorten the length of the study because all patients can then be assigned to the new treatment.

The advent of statistical procedures, such as the regression models of chapter 12, which can adjust the comparison of two treatments for differing distributions of other prognostic factors in the two treatment arms, has possibly made the use of historical controls more appealing. This is because randomization appears to be unnecessary as a mechanism for ensuring comparability of the treatment arms. The weak point in this reasoning is that absolute faith is being placed in the mathematical form of the statistical model and in the choice of prognostic factors. Changes in patients and patient care from one period to another may be quite subtle, but they may generate an apparent treatment effect because the proper adjustment for such changes is unknown.

Using data from the National Wilms' Tumor Study Group, *Farewell and D'Angio* [1981] examined these two approaches to treatment comparisons. In the first National Wilms' Tumor Study (NWTS-1), Group II and III patients were randomly assigned to three treatment groups – two single-drug chemotherapy regimens (A and B) and a double-drug regimen (C) which used both actinomycin-D and vincristine. The results of the study indicated that regimen C was the better treatment with respect to both relapse and survival. In the second National Wilms' Tumor Study (NWTS-2), regimen C was compared with a three-drug regimen (D) which added adriamycin. A total of 142 patients were entered into NWTS-1 on regimen C; from NWTS-2, data were available on 177 Group II and III patients who had received regimen D and on 179 patients who had received regimen C.

Two important prognostic factors for Wilms' tumor are histology (favorable and unfavorable) and nodal involvement. Other factors of lesser importance are age (> 2 years) and tumor weight (> 250 g). *Farewell and D'Angio* chose to analyze the response variable relapse-free survival using the relative risk regression model

$$d_j(t; \underline{x}) = d_{0j}(t) \exp(\Sigma b_i x_i)$$

discussed in chapter 12. In all the analyses described below, the effect of histology was accounted for by stratification and the remaining factors were included in $\underline{x}$, the vector of explanatory covariates.

Table 14.1. The results of two proportional hazards analyses of NWTS data: **(a)** using historical controls; **(b)** using concurrent controls

Covariate	Coefficient	Standard error	z-statistic
a Historical controls			
Regimen D	−0.21	0.29	0.72
Positive nodes	0.58	0.31	1.87
Tumor weight > 250 g	−0.10	0.45	0.22
Age > 2 years	0.44	0.39	1.13
b Concurrent controls			
Regimen D	−0.58	0.27	2.15
Positive nodes	0.88	0.28	3.14
Tumor weight > 250 g	0.16	0.43	0.37
Age > 2 years	0.27	0.37	0.73

Reproduced from: Farewell, V.T.; D'Angio, G.J.: A simulated study of historical controls using real data. Biometrics *37:* 169–176 (1981). With permission from the Biometric Society.

Table 14.1 presents the results of two separate analyses. The first analysis compares the relapse-free survival rates of the 177 patients receiving regimen D in NWTS-2 with the 142 patients receiving regimen C in NWTS-1. The second analysis is based only on NWTS-2 data and compares the 177 patients receiving regimen D with the 179 patients receiving regimen C. The first analysis, which is based on historical controls, indicates no beneficial effect from regimen D, whereas the analysis based on concurrent controls indicates a significant, beneficial effect. More extensive modelling did not alter these conclusions. A comparison of the relapse-free survival rates of the patients who received regimen C in the two studies did not reveal any significant treatment difference (p = 0.09).

The final decision concerning the superiority of regimen D relative to regimen C depends on many factors involved in total patient care, for example, short- and long-term complications caused by the therapies. Historical data should not be ignored, but in the NWTS a better basis for a decision was provided by using both past and concurrent information rather than historical data alone. In fact, the design of the third National Wilms' Tumor Study reflects a conclusion that some advantage for D, measured in disease-free survival, has been established, but there are questions about the potentially lethal, delayed cardiotoxicity of the regimen that remain to be answered. Therefore, NWTS-3 compares a modified, more intensive version of regimen C with a modified regimen D.

The results of a single trial are unlikely to resolve a controversy as involved as that of historical controls versus concurrent controls. This example does illustrate, however, some of the differences that could occur between the two types of studies.

The use of historical controls is often advocated, as in the NWTS, when a series of studies for treatment of a particular disease is being planned. The best treatment group in the most recent study becomes the control group for the succeeding study. Such an approach may be particularly prone to problems. By using the data from the best treatment in one study, the efficacy of that treatment will probably be overestimated; therefore, in a subsequent study, the results of an analysis which uses historical controls and one involving randomized controls could be different. To illustrate this principle, let us suppose that there is no real difference between two treatments, but in a particular trial one treatment, by chance, produces better results. If the same treatment is applied in a subsequent trial, it will probably generate poorer results than it did in the first trial. And even when there is a real difference between treatments, the danger of overestimating the efficacy of the better treatment is present.

Some research by *Sacks* et al. [1982] suggests that the use of any available historical data as a control for a new treatment can lead to overestimates of the new treatment's effectiveness. In a literature review, *Sacks* et al. found 8 randomized clinical trials and 21 trials which used historical information to compare surgical and medical treatment for coronary artery disease. Only one of the randomized clinical trials identified a significant difference in overall survival between the two treatment groups. Nearly all the trials based on historical controls found the surgical treatment to be better. Table 14.2, which is taken from *Sacks* et al. [1982], compares long-term survival in the 6 randomized and 9 historical trials which provided such data. The pooled historical trials show both a higher survival for surgical patients and a lower survival for medical patients. When the historical trial data are adjusted to have the same overall proportions of one-, two- and three-vessel disease as the randomized trials, the difference between the medical and surgical groups is decreased, but is still larger than the corresponding difference in the randomized trials. This adjustment was only possible for 6 of the historical trials.

Table 14.2. Pooled estimates of overall survival in clinical trials of medical versus surgical treatment of coronary artery disease [*Sacks* et al., 1982][1]

	Number of studies	Number of patients	Percent survival			
			1 year	2 years	3 years	4 years
Randomized trials	6	18,861				
Surgical			92.4	89.6	87.6	85.3
Medical			93.4	89.2	83.2	79.8
Historical trials	9	9,290				
Surgical			93.0	92.2	90.9	88.3
Medical			83.8	78.2	71.1	65.5
Surgical adjusted[2]			93.7	92.5	91.2	87.4
Medical adjusted[2]			88.2	82.2	70.9	67.7

[1] Reprinted by permission of The American Journal of Medicine *72:* 235 (1982).
[2] Adjusted to have the same proportions with one-, two- and three-vessel disease as the randomized trials.

Although we have not discussed all the issues involved in opting for a randomized clinical trial, we strongly suggest that the use of historical controls can be a potentially misleading approach to treatment comparisons. Other researchers are similarly convinced. This fact, and the evident scientific advantages of concurrent, randomized controls must be given serious consideration, together with the ethical issues, in designing clinical trials.

As a final historical comment, we note that the concept of randomized experiments was proposed in order to avoid the many problems which arise in the analysis of non-randomized data. These problems were aptly described by *George Yule* [1924], who was quoted by *Irwin* [1963] in his presidential address to the Royal Statistical Society:

'The unhappy statistician has to try to disentangle the effect from the ravelled skein with which he is presented. No easy matter this, very often, and a matter demanding not merely a knowledge of method, but all the best qualities that an investigator can possess – strong common sense, caution, reasoning power and imagination. And when he has come to his conclusion the statistician must not forget his caution: he should not be dogmatic. 'You can prove anything by statistics' is a common gibe. Its contrary is more nearly true – you can never prove anything by statistics. The statistician is dealing with the most complex cases of multiple causation. He may show the facts are in accordance with this hypothesis or that. But it is quite another thing to show all other possible hypotheses are excluded, and that the facts do not admit of any other interpretation than the particular one he may have in mind'.

14.4. Factorial Designs

The majority of clinical trials are designed, primarily, to answer a single question. This is often an unnecessary restriction on the design of a trial, especially for diseases which require multi-modal therapy.

For example, when the third National Wilms' Tumor Study was being designed, there were two questions of interest concerning Stage II, favorable histology, patients. One question concerned the chemotherapy comparison of two- and three-drug regimens which was mentioned in §14.3; the other was whether post-operative radiation was necessary for these patients. Since the number of cases of Wilms' tumor is small and the relapse-free survival rate is very high, two separate trials to address these questions were not feasible.

Both questions can be answered, however, in a factorial design. The schematic layout for the design is shown in Table 14.3. Patients are randomized among four regimens, and the sample size of the study need not be much larger than that required to answer either question separately. The radiation question is addressed by comparing regimen W to regimen X and regimen Y to regimen Z. The chemotherapy comparison is based on W versus Y and X versus Z. With this design, it is also possible to detect a synergistic (or antagonistic) interaction between the two modalities, although if such an effect is suspected, it might be necessary to increase the sample size somewhat.

We will not describe the details of analyzing such studies; nevertheless, factorial designs pose no major analytical problems. Therefore, if the flexibility of such a trial design is attractive, researchers should not be reluctant to consider using designs of this type.

Table 14.3. The factorial design for Stage II patients in the third National Wilms' Tumor Study

	No radiation	2,000 rads
Vincristine and actinomycin-D	Regimen W	Regimen X
Vincristine, actinomycin-D and adriamycin	Regimen Y	Regimen Z

Table 14.4. The overall probability of a significant test with repeated hypothesis testing [*McPherson, 1974*]

Nominal significance level	Number of repeat tests								
	1	2	3	4	5	10	25	50	200
0.01	0.01	0.018	0.024	0.029	0.033	0.047	0.070	0.088	0.126
0.05	0.05	0.083	0.107	0.126	0.142	0.193	0.266	0.320	0.424
0.10	0.10	0.160	0.202	0.234	0.260	0.342	0.449	0.524	0.652

Reprinted by permission of The New England Journal of Medicine *290:* 501 (1974).

14.5. Repeated Significance Testing

In chapter 13, we discussed the problem of multiple comparisons. A related problem in the analysis of clinical trials is known as repeated significance testing.

When a clinical trial is ongoing, it is common, and ethically necessary, to prepare interim analyses of the accrued data. If one treatment can be shown to be superior, then it is necessary to stop the trial so that all patients may receive the optimal treatment. Unfortunately, the more frequently the study data are examined, the more likely it is that a 'statistically significant' result will be observed.

Table 14.4, taken from *McPherson* [1974], illustrates this effect by showing the overall probability of observing a significant result at three nominal significance levels when a test is repeated differing numbers of times. Although this table is based on 'some fairly rigid technical assumptions' and may not be directly relevant to all clinical trials, it illustrates clearly that multiple tests at the same nominal significance level can be very misleading. For example, if we conduct ten analyses which test for a treatment difference at the nominal significance level of 0.05, the chance of falsely detecting a treatment difference is nearly 0.20, not 0.05.

There is a fair amount of statistical literature concerning formal trial designs which adjust for the effect of repeated significance testing; this area of research is known as sequential analysis. To a large extent, this predominantly theoretical work has had little effect on the actual design of medical trials. We believe that this is the case because the formalism does not yet

accurately reflect the conditions under which many medical trials are conducted. A formal significance test is often one of many components in the
decision to continue or stop a trial. Nevertheless, some of the more recent
research in sequential analysis has greater potential for application and
may yet affect the design of clinical trials.

The main purpose of this section has been to make the reader aware of
a frequently occurring problem in medical studies. A clinical trial should
not be stopped as soon as a significant result at the 5% level has been detected. When data are constantly re-examined, and updated, the advice of
a statistician should be sought before any major decisions are made on the
basis of an analysis which ignores the effect of repeated statistical testing.

14.6. Sequential Analysis

The conventional view of a clinical trial can be regarded as a 'fixed
sample design'. This means that a sample size is determined at the planning
stage, and that the trial results are analyzed once the specified sample size
has been achieved. However, as the previous section has indicated, the
usual monitoring of a clinical trial often makes it 'de facto' a sequential
experiment with repeated analyses over time. In this section, we give a brief
introduction to some actual sequential designs. Because of technical details
which we choose not to discuss, we recommend that a statistician be consulted before initiating a sequential trial. Nonetheless, we hope this section
will provide useful background material for interested readers.

Most sequential designs start with the supposition that the primary
comparison of the clinical trial can be represented by a test statistic. We
shall represent this statistic by Z to suggest that, under the null hypothesis
of no treatment difference, it is usually normally distributed with mean 0
and variance 1. For example, Z might be the usual ratio of the estimated
regression coefficient associated with treatment to its estimated standard
error. At any point in time during the trial, Z can be calculated.

The approach to sequential design advocated by *Whitehead* [1983] is to
consider what we might expect to see, if the null hypothesis is true, and if Z
was observed or calculated continuously over time. While this is clearly
impractical, it is an approach which leads to reasonable procedures that can
be slightly modified to reflect the usual monitoring strategy. The essential
characteristic of the design ensures that if there is no treatment difference,
the overall probability, for the complete trial, of concluding that the data

are not consistent with the null hypothesis is a specified significance level α. The value represented by α would often be the customary 5% level of significance. A decision that the data are inconsistent with the null hypothesis is frequently referred to as 'rejecting the null hypothesis'. Thus, in a sequential design of the type described above, the probability of rejecting the null hypothesis, on the basis of Z, sometime during the trial, is equal to α. By way of comparison, in a trial of fixed sample design a single significance test at level α is performed at the end of the trial. Since the technical details of *Whitehead's* approach are beyond the scope of this book, we will not discuss it further.

A second approach, known as group sequential designs, acknowledges that analyses will usually take place at specified times and presents a design based on a plan to perform a fixed number of analyses, say K, at distinct times. Group sequential designs which parallel the continuous procedures of *Whitehead* [1983] choose a testing significance level for the jth test which is the same for all tests and such that the overall probability of rejecting the null hypothesis, if it is true, is equal to α. Thus, for example, a design which involved four planned analyses and an overall significance level of 5% would perform a significance test at each analysis at a testing significance level of 0.018. Since

$$1-(1-0.018)^4 = 1-(0.982)^4$$
$$= 1-0.95 = 0.05,$$

the overall probability of rejecting the null hypothesis, if it is true, in any of the four tests is 0.05.

We are sympathetic to the arguments advanced by *Fleming* et al. [1984] that treatment differences observed in the early stages of a trial may occur for a variety of reasons, and that the primary purpose of a sequential design is to protect against unexpectedly large treatment differences. Therefore, *Fleming* et al. advocate using group sequential designs which preserve the sensitivity to late-occurring survival differences that a fixed sample design based on a single analysis would have. In addition, they argue that if the final analysis of a group sequential design is reached, then one would like to proceed, as much as possible, as if the preliminary analyses had not been done and a fixed sample design had been used.

To achieve these ends, *Fleming* et al. present designs in which the level of significance at which an intermediate analysis is performed increases as the trial progresses, and such that the testing level of significance for the final analysis is close to the overall level of α. Their proposal fulfills the

Table 14.5. Testing significance levels $\alpha_1, ..., \alpha_5$ for some group sequential designs

K	μ	α_1	α_2	α_3	α_4	α_5
2	0.1	0.00500	0.04806	–	–	–
	0.3	0.01500	0.04177	–	–	–
	0.5	0.02500	0.03355	–	–	–
3	0.1	0.00250	0.00296	0.04831	–	–
	0.3	0.00750	0.00936	0.04292	–	–
	0.5	0.01250	0.01606	0.03558	–	–
4	0.1	0.00167	0.00194	0.00233	0.04838	–
	0.3	0.00500	0.00612	0.00753	0.04342	–
	0.5	0.00833	0.01047	0.01306	0.03660	–
5	0.1	0.00128	0.00144	0.00164	0.00219	0.04806
	0.3	0.00379	0.00447	0.00527	0.00642	0.04319
	0.5	0.00634	0.00776	0.00931	0.01134	0.03691

The overall level of significance is 0.05, and 0.05 μ is the probability of terminating the trial early, if the null hypothesis is true, at any of the K analyses.
Adapted from *Fleming* et al. [1984]; it appears here with the kind permission of the publisher.

ethical requirement of protecting patients while not creating substantial additional difficulties in the data analysis. The designs are characterized by K, the number of planned analyses, α, the overall significance level, and by $\mu\alpha$, the probability of terminating the trial early if the null hypothesis is true. The fraction μ is, in some sense, the proportion of the overall probability of rejecting the null hypothesis which is used up prior to the final analysis. If we denote the testing levels of significance for the K analyses by $\alpha_1, \alpha_2, ..., \alpha_K$ then specifying μ is equivalent to specifying the ratio of α_K and α, i.e., $R = \alpha_K/\alpha$. This ratio indicates how close to the overall level α the final analysis is to be performed, and reflects the effect which the sequential nature of the design is allowed to have.

Table 14.5 presents a subset of the designs described in *Fleming* et al. [1984]. The table covers the cases specified by $\alpha = 0.05$, K = 2, 3, 4, and 5 and $\mu = 0.1, 0.3$ and 0.5. For example, if three analyses were planned and it was important to keep the ratio R high, i.e., $\mu = 0.1$ so that $R = \frac{0.04831}{0.05} = 0.97$, then the testing significance levels would be $\alpha_1 = 0.00250$, $\alpha_2 = 0.00296$ and $\alpha_3 = 0.04831$. On the other hand, if a more liberal stopping

Table 14.6. Anticipated results from the use of a sequential design proposed by *Fleming* et al. [1984] for a clinical trial of extensive stage small-cell lung cancer

Date	Total number of patients randomized to		Number of deaths observed	Testing significance level for early termination	Log-rank p-value observed
	regimen A	regimen B			
9/12/77	19	17	15	0.007	0.013
5/5/78	30	32	30	0.008	0.214
11/12/78	32	33	45	0.010	0.701
7/15/79	32	33	60	0.040	0.785

Adapted from *Fleming* et al. [1984]; it appears here with the kind permission of the publisher.

criterion was desirable, the design with $\mu = 0.5$ would result in testing significance levels of $\alpha_1 = 0.01250$, $\alpha_2 = 0.01606$ and $\alpha_3 = 0.03558$ with $R = 0.03558/0.05 = 0.71$.

Table 14.6 is abstracted from *Fleming* et al. and reports the results of a clinical trial of extensive stage small-cell lung cancer. Two chemotherapy regimens, denoted by A and B, were to be compared. Calculations based on a fixed sample design to compare death rates using the log-rank test suggest that the study would require about 60 deaths. The nature of these calculations is outlined in the next chapter. If we assume that $K = 4$ log-rank analyses are planned during the trial, one every 15 deaths, and if we also require $R = \alpha_4/\alpha = 0.8$, then the four testing significance levels which result are $\alpha_1 = 0.007$, $\alpha_2 = 0.008$, $\alpha_3 = 0.010$ and $\alpha_4 = 0.040$.

From Table 14.6 it can be seen that although there was a relatively large treatment difference early in the trial, this difference would not have been sufficient to stop the trial. Moreover, by the end of the trial no treatment difference was apparent.

This section is not intended to be a comprehensive treatment of the topic of sequential designs. Additional study of the subject, and consultation with a statistician, would be essential before embarking on a clinical trial which involves a sequential design. However, we do feel that the designs proposed by *Fleming* et al., which we have described, are consistent with the usual practice of clinical trials. Therefore, they may be of interest to some readers.

A Selected Bibliography

Breslow, N.: Perspectives on the statistician's role in cooperative clinical research. Cancer *41:* 326–332 (1978).

Brown, B.W.: The use of controls in the clinical evaluation of cancer therapies; in Proceedings of a symposium on statistical aspects of protocol design, pp. 161–180 (National Cancer Institute, Bethesda 1970).

Byar, D.P.; Simon, R.M.; Friedewald, W.T.; Schlesselman, J.J.; DeMets, D.L.; Ellenberg, J.H.; Gail, M.H.; Ware, J.H.: Randomized clinical trials. New Engl. J. Med. *295:* 74–80 (1976).

Chalmers, T.C.: Randomized clinical trials in surgery; in Varco, Delaney, Controversy in surgery, pp. 3–11 (Saunders, Philadelphia 1976).

Chalmers, T.C.; Block, J.B.; Lee, S.: Controlled studies in clinical cancer research. New Engl. J. Med. *287:* 75–78 (1972).

Cox, D.R.: Summary views: a statistician's perspective. Cancer Treat. Rep. *64:* 533–535 (1980).

Farewell, V.T.; D'Angio, G.J.: A simulated study of historical controls using real data. Biometrics *37:* 169–176 (1981).

Freireich, E.J.: The randomized clinical trial as an obstacle to clinical research; in Varco, Delaney, Controversy in surgery, vol. 2, pp. 5–12 (Saunders, Philadelphia 1983).

Gehan, E.A.; Freireich, E.J.: Non-randomized controls in cancer clinical trials. New Engl. J. Med. *290:* 198–203 (1974).

Peto, R.; Pike, M.C.; Armitage, P.; Breslow, N.E.; Cox, D.R.; Howard, S.V.; Mantel, N.; McPherson, K.; Peto, J.; Smith, P.G.: Design and analysis of randomized clinical trials requiring prolonged observation of each patient. I. Introduction and design. Br. J. Cancer *34:* 585–612 (1976).

Sacks, H.; Chalmers, T.C.; Smith, H.: Randomized versus historical controls for clinical trials. Am. J. Med. *72:* 233–240 (1982).

15 The Question of Sample Size

15.1. Introduction

In the preceding chapter, we briefly introduced a few of the important issues which arise in the design of clinical trials. The question of sample size is a technical consideration comprising one aspect of the general problem of design. Although, in general terms, it is difficult to specify how many subjects are required to make a clinical trial worthwhile, to embark on any study without considering the sample size which is adequate is unwise, and may even be unethical. It is not appreciated widely enough that failure to detect a treatment difference may often be related more to inadequate sample size than to the actual lack of a real difference between competing therapies. In the final analysis, studies with inadequate sample sizes serve only to confuse the issue of determining the most effective therapy.

Sample size calculations are frequently complicated; therefore, we do not intend to describe the actual details in depth. Instead, we propose to highlight those aspects of the subject which are common to all situations, describing these features in non-technical terms. To illustrate the basic concepts in a more practical setting, we discuss the determination of appropriate sample sizes for two different hypothetical studies in §15.3. And, in the final section of the chapter, we point out some of the hazards associated with small clinical trials.

15.2. General Aspects of Sample Size Calculations

It is important to realize, right from the start, that sample size calculations will always be approximate. It is clearly impossible to predict the exact outcome of any particular clinical trial or laboratory experiment. Nevertheless, the importance of sample size calculations is demonstrated by the fact that they provide information about two important design questions:

(1) How many subjects should participate in the intended experiment?

(2) Is this study worth doing if only n subjects (a fixed number) participate?

Clearly, both questions enable an investigator to evaluate the study or experiment critically, and to decide whether to proceed as planned, or perhaps to revise the overall design. In certain cases, the wisest decision may be not to initiate the study because the likelihood of demonstrating the desired effect, using the available resources of personnel, funds and participants, is very small.

In chapter 13 we suggested that, in most studies, there will be a primary question which the researchers want to investigate. The calculations concerning sample size depend on this primary question and the way in which it is to be answered. Therefore, in order to answer either of the two questions posed above, an investigator needs to decide what sort of data will be collected and how these data are to be analyzed. These choices need not be rigidly determined; indeed, they never can be since almost every study will involve some unexpected features. All the same, since sample size calculations depend on the proposed method of analysis, some tentative assumptions are necessary. Already, it should be obvious to the reader why sample size calculations are only approximate.

For the sake of illustration, let us suppose that a clinical trial is being planned. The chief purpose of the trial is to compare the effectiveness of an experimental treatment with the current standard procedure, called the control treatment. Without being too specific, we can state that an answer to the primary question can be expressed in terms of a clinically relevant treatment difference. For example, this difference might be the reduction in mortality experienced by patients receiving the experimental treatment. The study is being conducted to determine the degree to which the results are consistent with the null hypothesis of no treatment difference. Either a treatment difference will be demonstrated, or the data will be judged consistent with the null hypothesis.

An additional degree of artificiality is introduced into sample size calculations by the convention that failure to reject the null hypothesis is equivalent to concluding that the null hypothesis is true. This convention is inappropriate at the time of analysis, but convenient at the design stage.

The true situation in the study population concerning the null hypothesis, H_0, can never be known for certain. Also, with respect to the true situation, the researcher's final conclusions regarding the treatment difference may be correct or wrong. Table 15.1a concisely sums up the framework within which sample size calculations are undertaken.

In two of the four cases that could arise, the researcher will reach a correct conclusion. However, in the remaining two cases the researcher will be wrong, having reached either a false positive or a false negative conclusion. Traditionally, statisticians have called these erroneous outcomes Type I and Type II errors, and have represented the probabilities of these two outcomes by α and β, respectively (see Table 15.1b). In our view, the terms false positive and false negative are more informative in the medical research setting.

If no treatment difference exists, then α is simply the probability of obtaining an unlikely outcome in that situation and therefore deciding that the data contradict the null hypothesis. This probability is precisely the significance level of the data with respect to H_0, i.e., the p-value. The value of α which the investigator uses to conclude whether H_0 is true or false is usually regarded as fixed in advance.

If a real treatment difference exists, i.e., if H_0 is false, the probability that the investigator will correctly conclude that this is so is $1-\beta$ (see Table 15.1b). This probability depends largely on N, the total sample size, but also on the actual magnitude of the treatment difference. The reason for this dependence on total sample size is fairly simple. A larger sample contains more information about characteristics which are of interest, and hence facilitates more precise estimation of the true situation that obtains in the study population. Therefore, by increasing the sample size, we increase our ability to detect any real treatment difference which exists. This increased ability to determine whether H_0 is true or false is translated into an increased probability, $1-\beta$, that a correct conclusion will be reached when H_0 is false. Since $(1-\beta) + \beta = 1$, if $(1-\beta)$ increases, then the false negative probability, β, necessarily decreases. Therefore, increasing the sample size can also be viewed as a means of decreasing the false negative rate when a real treatment difference exists.

We are now in a position to state, in precise terms, the two questions about any study which sample size calculations will answer:

(1) If the probability of a false positive conclusion is fixed at α, what total sample size, N, is required to ensure that the probability of detecting a clinically relevant difference of given magnitude δ is $1-\beta$?

(2) If the probability of a false positive conclusion is fixed at α, and a specific sample size, N, is employed, what is the probability, $1-\beta$, that the study will detect a clinically relevant difference of given magnitude δ?

Table 15.1. The hypothetical framework of sample size calculations: **(a)** correct and erroneous conclusions; **(b)** probabilities of correct and erroneous conclusions

True situation	Investigator's conclusion	
	H_0 True	H_0 False
a Correct and erroneous conclusions		
H_0 True	correct conclusion	false positive (Type I error)
H_0 False	false negative (Type II error)	correct conclusion
b Probabilities of correct and erroneous conclusions		
H_0 True	$1-\alpha$	α
H_0 False	β	$1-\beta$

Notice that to answer the first question we must specify sample sizes, N, which correspond to prescribed triples of α, δ and $1-\beta$. On the other hand, to answer the second question we must determine values of $1-\beta$ which correspond to specific values of α, δ and N. In either case, the answer would not be a single value, but rather a table, or perhaps a graph, of sample sizes, N, or probabilities, $1-\beta$.

Of course, other considerations besides the method of evaluation and the clinically relevant treatment difference will affect the determination of adequate sample size. These include the relative sizes of the treatment groups, possible dropout rates in these groups and the thorny problem of treatment noncompliance. Unfortunately, a researcher may have no effective means of controlling some of these factors which can seriously affect the anticipated outcome of the study. In addition, any failure to observe uniform standards in evaluating patient characteristics or treatment outcomes may increase overall variability in the study. The inevitable consequence will be a reduced ability to detect any real treatment difference which exists.

It is beyond the scope of this book to give many of the details involved in performing sample size calculations. The time spent consulting a statistician, or undertaking additional reading, on this aspect of study design will be seen, we hope, as time well spent. To prepare the reader for such activities, in the following section we discuss two hypothetical studies and describe the aspects of each which would be considered in evaluating the required sample size.

Comments:

(a) Since α and β both represent probabilities of making an erroneous decision, in the best of all possible worlds we would like both α and β to be close to zero. Unfortunately, if α is decreased without changing the total sample size, N, then β necessarily increases. Conversely, if β must decrease without changing N, then α necessarily increases. Only by increasing the sample size can a simultaneous reduction in both α and β be achieved.

(b) Typically, the value of α is fixed by the experimenter, since α is the p-value at which the study outcome will be regarded as statistically significant. In this case, β will decrease as the total sample size increases. The decision regarding an adequate sample size for a given study will necessarily be a compromise, balancing what can be achieved, statistically, with a sample size that is practical.

(c) The probability, 1–β, of detecting a specified difference, δ, is called the power of the study. A powerful study is one with a high probability of detecting an important treatment difference. It has been proposed that if a study fails to reject the null hypothesis, then it is important to state the power of the study. Although this proposal would aid in the interpretation of a study's conclusions, we believe it is an inappropriate use of power calculations. Sample size (or power) calculations are relevant to study design, not analysis. At the analysis stage, the results of significance tests and statistical estimation are relevant. If a confidence interval is provided for an estimated treatment difference, then power calculations will furnish no additional information. In addition, the assumptions inherent in power calculations are generally more restrictive than those required at the analysis stage.

15.3. Two Examples of Sample Size Calculations

15.3.1. A Comparison of Proportions

Several researchers are proposing to conduct a clinical trial to evaluate the effectiveness of the β-blocker, metoprolol, in reducing mortality following acute myocardial infarction. It has been decided that the outcome of interest in the study is to be death within 90 days of the initial attack. While many of the details of the study protocol have yet to be determined, the study collaborators have decided to conduct a double-blind, randomized, controlled trial using a suitable placebo. With respect to the primary purpose of the study, the data will be analyzed using the methods for 2×2 contingency tables.

Effectively, the study is designed to compare the proportions of deaths within 90 days (90-day mortality rates) observed in the two study groups. The researchers anticipate that the mortality rate for metoprolol will be significantly lower than the corresponding value for the placebo. How large should the total sample size for the study be?

In order to carry out sample size calculations, the consulting statistician needs some additional details regarding the study. The researchers will have to estimate the mortality rate which they expect to observe in the placebo group; in addition, the clinically relevant difference between the two mortality rates which they want to be able to detect is also needed. If unequal group sizes are to be used, the fraction that each group represents of the total sample size must be specified. Finally, the investigators must determine the value of α, the probability of a false positive result, which they are willing to accept. Once these items have been specified, the statistician will be able to generate a table of sample sizes and the corresponding values of β, the probability of a false negative result.

After some discussion, the researchers report that the expected mortality rate in the placebo group is about 0.20 and the clinically relevant difference is a reduction in the mortality rate to 0.10 or less. This is the treatment difference that they want to be able to detect. The study participants will be randomized in equal numbers to the two treatments and the traditional α-value of 0.05, i.e., $p = 0.05$, will be used to evaluate the statistical significance of the study.

In many cases, a statistician is able to refer to statistical tables for sample size calculations which help to answer a client's query. For the particular situation described above, Table 15.2a, which indicates the required net total sample size, N, and the corresponding probability of a false negative, β, might be prepared.

Notice that the calculations specify net total sample size. If provision is to be made for patient dropout and treatment noncompliance, the necessary sample sizes will be larger than those indicated in the table.

15.3.2. An Analysis of Survival Data

In this hypothetical study, the researcher is proposing to conduct an experiment concerned with death due to vaginal cancer in rats insulted with the carcinogen DMBA. Two groups of equal size will have differing pretreatment regimens. The rats will be observed for a specified period. The primary purpose of the study is to determine whether survival depends on the pretreatment regimen.

Table 15.2. Two sample size tables for hypothetical studies: (a) comparing proportions; (b) analyzing survival data

a Comparing proportions

N	100	200	300	400	500	600	700
β	0.71	0.48	0.31	0.19	0.11	0.06	0.04

b Analyzing survival data

Survival rate in the poorer group at the time of analysis	Survival advantage enjoyed by the better group	
	0.05	0.10
0.05	497 (661)[1]	174 (232)
0.10	963 (1289)	295 (395)
0.15	1415 (1894)	406 (544)

[1] Sample size required to yield β = 0.20 (0.10).

Observations on rats which die of causes unrelated to the application of the carcinogen and are free of tumor at death, or rats which simply have not developed tumor at the time of data analysis will be censored observations on the time of death from vaginal cancer. To analyze the experimental data, a log-rank test (see chapter 7) for the treatment difference will be used.

In order to prepare some sample size tables for this particular study the following are required: the proportion of rats in each treatment group which are likely to be free of tumor at the time the experimenter decides to terminate the experiment and α, the probability of a false positive result which will be used to determine the statistical significance of the log-rank test. With some difficulty, the investigator eventually estimates that the survival rates in the two groups at the time of analysis are likely to range from 0.05 to 0.15 for the poorer group, with the other treatment group possibly enjoying an advantage of 0.05 to 0.10. The usual probability of a false positive conclusion, namely α = 0.05, will be used to evaluate the log-rank test.

Based on these values and sample size tables for the log-rank test produced by *Freedman* [1982], the statistician draws up Table 15.2b. Entries in the table specify the total sample size which is required to yield 0.20 probability of reaching a false negative conclusion with respect to the indicated survival advantage (treatment difference). The numbers in parentheses correspond to a false negative probability level of 0.10.

The values given in the table presuppose that all rats either die of vaginal cancer or are observed free of tumor at the time of analysis. If an appreciable fraction of the original experimental group are likely to yield censored observations prior to the termination of the experiment, then the numbers given in Table 15.2b will need to be increased to adjust for this loss in information regarding death due to vaginal cancer.

In both of the examples we have just considered, the 'answer' regarding sample size has not been a single number, but rather a table of values. This method of presentation highlights several of the features of sample size calculations which we discussed in §15.2. For example, sample size calculations are, by nature, approximate, since the results depend on tentative assumptions regarding the expected outcome of the study. Moreover, the actual sample size which a researcher uses will inevitably be a compromise between the values of α and β which are acceptable, and the cost of the study in terms of resources and time per participant. More important still, sample size calculations can convince researchers that when patient numbers are too limited, certain studies should be concluded before they begin.

15.4. Some Hazards of Small Studies

In preceding sections of this chapter we have suggested, without justification, that studies which involve only a small number of participants may not be worth doing. In this final section, we intend to provide the reader with sound reasons to be wary of conclusions which are derived from small experiments or clinical trials.

As a starting point, let us consider the following hypothetical situation which is discussed in *Pocock* [1983]. Suppose the response rate for the standard treatment of a disease is 0.30. A number of new drugs are being developed and require evaluation in carefully-conducted clinical trials. Of course, not all the drugs will be more effective than the standard treatment. In fact, we will assume that 80% are no better than the standard treatment. The remaining 20% of new drugs will achieve a response rate of 0.50, and therefore represent a major advance in the treatment of the disease. The chief purpose of each clinical trial which may be held is to determine whether the drug being tested belongs to this latter category.

Table 15.3. Details of hypothetical clinical trials of five sizes illustrating some hazards of small studies

Size of trial	True response rates (experimental – standard)	Number of trials worldwide	Expected number of statistically significant trials (p ≤ 0.05)	Percentage expected of true positives detected	Ratio of expected false positives to expected true positives
400	0.30–0.30	40	2	–	0.20
	0.50–0.30	10	9.9	99	
200	0.30–0.30	80	4	–	0.22
	0.50–0.30	20	17.9	90	
100	0.30–0.30	160	8	–	0.30
	0.50–0.30	40	26.4	66	
50	0.30–0.30	320	16	–	0.47
	0.50–0.30	80	34.0	43	
25	0.30–0.30	640	32	–	0.74
	0.50–0.30	160	43.0	27	

A number of clinical trials are held, worldwide, and in each trial one new drug is evaluated relative to the standard treatment. All trials are of the same total size, and the value of α, the probability of a false positive conclusion if the null hypothesis of no treatment difference is true, is the conventional 0.05. Each trial will be summarized as a 2×2 contingency table and analyzed accordingly.

The situation we have just outlined is admittedly simplistic. Nevertheless, we believe it can illustrate two of the major problems associated with small studies of any kind. Table 15.3 summarizes the expected outcome of the situation we have described for clinical trials of five different sizes – 400, 200, 100, 50 and 25 participants. For each of these five situations, a total of 20,000 participants are involved, worldwide.

The most important columns in Table 15.3 are the latter three; these indicate the expected number of trials which would be statistically significant ($p \leq 0.05$), the percentage expected of true positives that would be detected and the ratio of expected false positive to expected true positive trials. Notice, first, that as the trial size decreases from 400 to 25, the expected true positives detected decreases from 99 to 27%. Thus, trials involving few participants are clearly less capable of identifying the effective drugs than larger trials. Moreover, as trial size decreases, the ratio of expected false positive conclusions to expected true positives increases from 0.20 to 0.74. This reflects the fact that, since the value of α is usually fixed, a large number of small trials increases the likelihood that a positive conclusion is a false one.

But there are other problems which could easily arise if a particular study were to involve only a limited number of subjects. We have argued, in chapter 14, that randomization is advisable whenever its use is ethically defensible. To a statistician, randomization in a clinical trial is rather like the premium which a home owner pays annually for fire insurance coverage. If an important factor happens to be overlooked, inadvertently or unconsciously, during the planning of a certain trial, randomization should ensure that its effect is roughly similar in all treatment groups. However, the effectiveness of randomization depends on total sample size; randomizing a large number of participants is more likely to achieve the intended result.

Our final comment regarding the hazards of small studies concerns stratification. If a trial or experiment involves only a few participants, there will be little possibility of doing a stratified analysis, even if this is necessary. We have indicated elsewhere that stratification can be a very useful technique. However, if each stratum is likely to contain only a few subjects, there is little point in stratifying the data. Large experiments or clinical trials make stratification more feasible.

Our discussion of the hazards of small studies has not been exhaustive. Nevertheless, we hope that the need for a cautious interpretation of such studies has been demonstrated. Some years ago, a number of countries began to require that cigarette packages should bear a warning message for users. Perhaps small studies deserve to be similarly distinguished.

16 Epidemiological Applications

16.1. Introduction

Lilienfeld and Lilienfeld [1980] begin their text 'Foundations of Epidemiology' with the statement: 'Epidemiology is concerned with the pattern of disease occurrence in human populations and of the factors that influence these patterns.' In previous chapters we have concentrated on clinical data related primarily to disease outcome. Here we attempt to provide a brief introduction to the study of disease incidence, and illustrate how some of the statistical methods which we have discussed can be applied in various epidemiological studies.

16.2. Epidemiological Studies

The cohort study is the simplest approach to the study of disease incidence. A cohort, which is a random sample of a large population, is monitored for a fixed period of time in order to observe disease incidence. Important characteristics of each individual cohort member are ascertained at the start of the study and during the period of follow-up. This information is used to identify the explanatory variables or 'risk factors' which are related to disease incidence. Thus, risk factors are measured prospectively, that is, before the occurrence of disease. The cohort study also provides a direct estimate of the rate of disease incidence in the population subgroups which are defined by the explanatory variables. Section 16.3 describes, in considerable detail, the analysis of a cohort study which uses the method of proportional hazards regression that was introduced in chapter 12.

A special case of cohort data is population-based, cause-specific incidence and mortality data which are routinely collected for surveillance purposes in many parts of the world. These data are usually stratified by year, age at death (or incidence) and sex and have been used to study geographic and temporal variations in disease. In certain instances, aggregate data on explanatory variables such as fat consumption or smoking habits may also be available for incorporation into the analysis of these vital data.

For many diseases, the collection of cohort data is both time-consuming and expensive. Therefore, one of the most important study designs in epidemiology is the case-control study. This design involves the selection of a random sample of incident cases of the study disease in a defined population during a specified case accession period. Corresponding comparison individuals (the controls) are randomly selected from those members of the same population, or a specified subset of it, who are disease-free during the case accession period. Information on the values of explanatory variables during the time period prior to case or control ascertainment is obtained at the time of ascertainment. These retrospective data are usually subject to more error in measurement than the prospective data of the cohort study; however, a case-control study can be completed in a much shorter period of time. The case-control design facilitates comparisons of disease rates in different subsets of the study population but, since the number of cases and controls sampled is fixed by the design, it cannot provide an estimate of the actual disease rates. An important variation in case-control designs involves the degree of matching of cases to controls, particularly with respect to primary time variables such as subject age. In §16.4 we present an example of a case-control study in which logistic regression is used to analyze the data.

16.3. Relative Risk Models

In chapter 12, we introduced proportional hazards regression as a method for modelling a death rate function. This same method can also be used to model the rate of disease incidence. If we denote the disease incidence rate at time t by r(t), then we can rewrite equation (12.1) as

$$\log\{r(t;\underline{x})\} = \log\{r_0(t)\} + \sum_{i=1}^{k} b_i x_i, \tag{16.1}$$

where $\underline{x} = \{x_1, x_2, \ldots, x_k\}$ refers to a set of explanatory variables to be related to the incidence rate. The function $r_0(t)$ represents the disease incidence rate at time t for an individual whose explanatory variables are all equal to zero.

To illustrate how the regression model (16.1) can be used in epidemiology, consider the cohort study reported by *Prentice* et al. [1982]. This cohort study was based on nearly 20,000 residents of Hiroshima and Nagasaki,

identified by population census, and actively followed by the Radiation
Effects Research Foundation from 1958. Information concerning systolic
and diastolic blood pressure as well as a number of other cardiovascular
disease risk factors, was obtained during biennial examinations. During the
period 1958–1974, 16,711 subjects were examined at least once. In total,
108 incident cases of cerebral hemorrhage, 469 incident cases of cerebral
infarction and 218 incident cases of coronary heart disease were observed
during follow-up. The determination of the relative importance of systolic
and diastolic blood pressure as risk indicators for these three major cardiovascular disease categories was a primary objective of the analysis of these
data. The time variable t was defined to be the examination cycle (i.e., t = 1
in 1958–1960, t = 2 in 1960–1962, etc.). The use of this discrete time scale
introduces some minor technical issues which need not concern us here.

Two generalizations of model (16.1) which were introduced in chapter
12 are of particular importance to the application of the model to cohort
studies. Frequently, there are key variables for which the principal comparison in the analysis must be adjusted. For example, in the study of blood
pressure and cardiovascular disease it is important to adjust for the explanatory variables age and sex. A very general adjustment is possible through
the stratified version of Cox's regression model, for which the defining
equation is

$$\log\{r_j(t; \underline{x})\} = \log\{r_{j0}(t)\} + \sum_{i=1}^{k} b_i x_i, \quad j = 1, \ldots, J. \tag{16.2}$$

Equation (16.2) specifies models for J separate strata, each of which has an
unspecified 'baseline' incidence rate $r_{j0}(t)$, where j indexes the strata. As in
the lymphoma example discussed in §12.3, the regression coefficients are
assumed to be the same in all strata. *Prentice* et al. [1982] used 32 strata
defined on the basis of sex and 16 five-year age categories.

The second generalization of model (16.1) involves the use of time-
dependent covariates. In this case the equation for the analysis model is

$$\log\{r_j[t; \underline{x}(t)]\} = \log\{r_{j0}(t)\} + \sum_{i=1}^{k} b_i x_i(t), \quad j = 1, \ldots, J. \tag{16.3}$$

In their analysis of the cohort data, *Prentice* et al. used blood pressure measurements at examinations undertaken before time t as covariates. Thus, for
example, Table 16.1 presents regression coefficients for a covariate vector,
$\underline{X}(t) = \{S(t-1), D(t-1)\}$, which represents the systolic and diastolic blood

Table 16.1. The results of a relative risk regression analysis of cardiovascular disease incidence in relation to previous examination cycle systolic and diastolic blood pressure measurements; the analyses stratify on age and sex

Regression variable	Cerebral hemorrhage $\hat{b}^a$ ($\times 10^2$)	Cerebral infarction $\hat{b}$ ($\times 10^2$)	Coronary heart disease $\hat{b}$ ($\times 10^2$)
S(t−1)	0.58 (0.30)[b]	1.77 (<0.0001)	1.15 (0.003)
D(t−1)	5.48 (<0.0001)	0.46 (0.36)	−0.46 (0.56)
Cases	92	406	187

[a] The estimated regression coefficients, $\hat{b}$, are maximum partial likelihood estimates.
[b] The values in parentheses are significance levels for testing the hypothesis b = 0.
Adapted from: Prentice, R.L. et al.: Serial blood pressure measurements and cardiovascular disease in a Japanese cohort. American Journal of Epidemiology *116:* 1–28 (1982). It appears here with the permission of the publisher.

pressure measurements, respectively, in examination cycle t−1. The table includes the corresponding significance levels for testing the hypothesis $b_i = 0$. Separate analyses are presented for each cardiovascular disease classification. The incidence of other disease classifications is regarded as censoring in each analysis. This is consistent with the assumption that the overall risk of cardiovascular disease is the sum of the three separate risks.

In Table 16.1, the diastolic blood pressure during the previous examination cycle is the important disease risk predictor for cerebral hemorrhage, whereas the corresponding systolic blood pressure is the more important predictor for cerebral infarction and for coronary heart disease. From Table 16.1, the estimated risk of cerebral hemorrhage for an individual with a diastolic blood pressure of 100 is

$$\exp\{0.0548(100-80)\} = 2.99$$

times that of an individual whose diastolic pressure is 80. Relative risks comparing any two individuals can be calculated in a similar way for each of the disease classifications.

The assumption that the blood pressure readings during the previous examination cycle are indeed the important predictors can be tested by

Table 16.2. The results of a relative risk regression analysis of cardiovascular disease incidence in relation to blood pressure measurements from the three preceding examination cycles; the analyses stratify on age and sex

Regression variable	Cerebral hemorrhage $\hat{b}^a$ ($\times 10^2$)	Cerebral infarction $\hat{b}$ ($\times 10^2$)	Coronary heart disease $\hat{b}$ ($\times 10^2$)
S(t–1)	–	1.13 (0.001)	–1.06 (0.06)
D(t–1)	3.23 (0.01)[b]	–	–
S(t–2)	–	0.80 (0.03)	1.46 (0.007)
D(t–2)	–1.07 (0.45)	–	–
S(t–3)	–	0.35 (0.30)	0.64 (0.22)
D(t–3)	4.77 (<0.0001)	–	–
Cases	48	207	97

[a] The estimated regression coefficients, $\hat{b}$, are maximum partial likelihood estimates.
[b] The values in parentheses are significance levels for testing the hypothesis b = 0.
Adapted from: Prentice, R.L. et al.: Serial blood pressure measurements and cardiovascular disease in a Japanese cohort. American Journal of Epidemiology *116:* 1–28 (1982). It appears here with the permission of the publisher.

defining new regression vectors $\underline{X}(t) = \{D(t–1), D(t–2), D(t–3)\}$ for the cerebral hemorrhage analysis and $\underline{X}(t) = \{S(t–1), S(t–2), S(t–3)\}$ for cerebral infarction and coronary heart disease. For a subject to contribute to these analyses at an incidence time t, all three previous biennial examinations must have been attended; therefore, the analyses presented in Table 16.2 involve fewer cases than the results reported in Table 16.1. The more extensive analysis presented in Table 16.2 suggests that the most recent systolic blood pressure measurement, S(t–1), is strongly associated with the risk of cerebral infarction, while the next most recent, S(t–2), shows a much weaker association. On the other hand, after adjusting for the levels of systolic blood pressure in the two preceding cycles, a recent elevated systolic blood pressure measurement is negatively associated, although marginally, with the risk of coronary heart disease. One possible explanation for this result would be the suggestion that hypertensive medication achieves blood pressure control without a corresponding reduction in coronary heart disease risk. The analysis for cerebral hemorrhage indicates that both elevated diastolic blood pressure and the duration of elevation are strongly related to the incidence of cerebral hemorrhage.

Tables 16.1 and 16.2 illustrate a complex application of the proportional hazards regression model in the analysis of cohort data. By discussing this example, we have tried to illustrate some of the possibilities for analysis which use of this model facilitates. There are a number of issues which arise in the analysis of cohort data via relative risk regression models which are beyond the scope of this book. In our view, however, these models represent a natural choice for the analysis of epidemiological cohort studies. We hope it is also clear that careful thought must be given to the form of a regression model that is used to analyze epidemiological data, and to the interpretation of the results.

16.4. Odds Ratio Models

In this section we consider the case-control study reported by *Weiss* et al. [1979]. This study identified and interviewed 322 cases of endometrial cancer occurring among white women in western Washington between January 1975 and April 1976. A random sample of 288 white women in the same age range were interviewed as controls. The interviews were used to obtain information on prior hormone use, particularly postmenopausal estrogen use, and on known risk factors for endometrial cancer.

Let Y be a binary variable which distinguishes cases (Y = 1) from controls (Y = 0). Then Y corresponds to the event of endometrial cancer incidence during the study period. If we also define a binary explanatory variable X which is equal to 0 unless a woman has used post-menopausal estrogens for more than one year (X = 1), then we require a statistical model which relates Y to X. A natural choice in this instance is the binary logistic regression model which was introduced in chapter 11. In terms of Y and X, the defining equation for this model is

$$\log \left\{ \frac{\Pr(Y = 1 \mid x)}{1 - \Pr(Y = 1 \mid x)} \right\} = a + bx. \tag{16.4}$$

As we indicated in § 11.3, e^b is the odds ratio which compares the odds of being a case for a woman using estrogen to the same odds for a non-user. The probability of cancer incidence for a non-user is equal to $\exp(a)/\{1 + \exp(a)\}$.

In § 16.2 we noted that, because the proportions of cases and controls are fixed by the study design, it is impossible to estimate the probability of cancer incidence, which depends on the parameter a, from a case-control study. Nevertheless, if case-control data are analyzed using a model like equation (16.4), then although the estimate of a has no practical value, the estimation of odds ratio parameters such as b can proceed in the usual fashion and provides valid estimates of odds ratios in the population under study. The justification for this claim is beyond the scope of this book, but if readers are willing to accept it at face value, we can proceed with an illustration of how logistic regression models can be used to analyze case-control studies.

In § 16.2 we mentioned the importance of age and the possible matching of cases and controls on age in case-control studies. Chapter 5 shows, in the context of 2×2 tables, that matching is a special case of stratification. In particular, pair matching, i.e., selecting one specific control for each case, corresponds to the use of strata of size two. Section 11.3 introduced the stratified version of a logistic regression model in the special case of two strata. A more general version of this stratified model is specified by the equation

$$\log\left\{\frac{\Pr(Y = 1 \mid \underline{x})}{1 - \Pr(Y = 1 \mid \underline{x})}\right\} = a_j + \sum_{i=1}^{k} b_i x_i, \quad j = 1, \ldots, J \qquad (16.5)$$

where j indexes the strata and the b_i's are the logarithms of odds ratios associated with the covariates in $\underline{X} = \{X_1, X_2, \ldots, X_k\}$. As was the case in § 11.3, the b_i's are assumed to be the same for each stratum.

Table 16.3 presents an analysis of the data reported by *Weiss* et al. [1979] when cases and controls are grouped in strata defined by one-year age intervals. The design of a case-control study usually includes some degree of matching on age; this ensures moderate balance between cases and controls in age-defined strata. Stratification on one-year age intervals is not always possible, but most studies would likely support strata based on five-year age intervals. With these one-year age intervals and women aged 50–74 years, problems would arise if we tried to estimate all 24 of the a_j's. The possibility of problems like this, and a method for avoiding them, was alluded to in

Table 16.3. The results of an odds ratio regression analysis of endometrial cancer incidence in relation to exposure to exogenous estrogens and other factors; the analysis stratifies on baseline age

Risk factor	Regression variable	Definition	$\hat{b}$	SE[a]	Significance level[b]
Estrogen use	X_1	1 if duration of use between 1 and 8 years; 0 otherwise	1.37	0.24	<0.0001
	X_2	1 if duration of use 8 years or greater; 0 otherwise	2.60	0.25	<0.0001
Obesity	X_3	1 if weight greater than 160 lbs; 0 otherwise	0.50	0.25	0.04
Hypertension	X_4	1 if history of high blood pressure; 0 otherwise	0.42	0.21	0.05
Parity	X_5	1 if number of children 2 or greater; 0 otherwise	0.81	0.21	0.0001

[a] Estimated standard error of $\hat{b}$.
[b] Estimated significance level for testing the hypothesis b = 0.

§11.3. Thus, Table 16.3 is based on a conditional analysis of model (16.5). This method of analysis adjusts for the stratification, but provides estimates of the b_i's without having to estimate the a_j's. We will not explain how a conditional analysis is carried out, but simply assure the reader that it does not alter the interpretation of the estimated b_i's which was presented in chapter 11.

The regression vector, $\underline{X}$, for each subject in the case-control study of endometrial cancer includes a binary variable, X_1, which is equal to 0 unless the subject had a duration of use of exogenous estrogen of between 1 and 8 years ($X_1 = 1$), a secondary variable, X_2, which is equal to 0 unless the subject had a duration of estrogen use in excess of 8 years ($X_2 = 1$), and additional indicator variables for obesity, hypertension and parity. On the basis of calculations which were outlined in §11.3, we conclude that estrogen use of between 1 and 8 years is associated with an estimated odds ratio for endometrial cancer of exp(1.37) = 3.94; the associated 95% confidence interval for the odds ratio is (2.46, 6.30). The corresponding estimate of the odds ratio and confidence interval associated with 8 years or more of estrogen use are exp(2.60) = 13.46 and (8.25, 21.98), respectively.

16.5. Confounding and Effect Modification

In the epidemiological literature, the terms confounding factor and effect modifying factor receive considerable attention. An epidemiological study is frequently designed to investigate a particular risk factor for a disease, and it is common practice to refer to this risk factor as an exposure variable, i.e., exposure to some additional risk. A confounding factor is commonly considered to be a variable which is related to both disease and exposure. Variables which have this property are discussed in §5.2 and will tend to bias any estimation of the relationship between disease and exposure. An effect modifying factor is a variable which may change the strength of the relationship between disease and exposure. The odds ratio, which associates exposure and disease, would vary with the level of an effect modifying variable. Confounding variables, and to a lesser extent effect modifying variables, are treated somewhat differently than exposure variables of direct interest because the former tend to be factors which are known to be related to disease. Therefore, it is necessary to adjust for confounding and effect modifying factors in any discussion of new risk factors. Although in formal statistical procedures this distinction between variables is not made, it can be an important practical question. Consequently, we propose to indicate how these concepts can be viewed in the context of regression models for case-control studies.

The analysis of epidemiological data using regression models like (16.3) and (16.5) will only identify something we choose to call 'potential' confounding variables. This is because the interrelation of the covariates is irrelevant in such an approach. Thus, the relationship between exposure and a potential confounding variable is never explored. Provided that the regression model is an adequate description of the data, its use will prevent a variable which is confounding in the common epidemiological sense from biasing the estimation of the odds ratio.

Effect-modification in a logistic regression model corresponds to something called an interaction effect in the statistical literature. Section 11.5 contains a brief discussion of the notion of interaction in the context of a

Table 16.4. The results of an odds ratio regression analysis of endometrial cancer incidence incorporating interaction terms for hypertension and estrogen use (cf. Table 16.3); the analysis stratifies on baseline age

Risk factor	Regression variable	Definition	$\hat{b}$	SE[a]	Significance level[b]
Estrogen use	X_1	1 if duration of use between 1 and 8 years; 0 otherwise	1.78	0.37	<0.0001
	X_2	1 if duration of use 8 years or greater; 0 otherwise	2.40	0.35	<0.0001
Obesity	X_3	1 if weight greater than 160 lbs; 0 otherwise	0.75	0.33	0.02
Hypertension	X_4	1 if history of high blood pressure; 0 otherwise	0.60	0.31	0.05
Parity	X_5	1 if number of children 2 or greater; 0 otherwise	0.58	0.31	0.06
Interaction terms	X_1X_4	1 if both X_1 and X_4 equal 1; 0 otherwise	−1.04	0.50	0.04
	X_2X_4	1 if both X_2 and X_4 equal 1; 0 otherwise	0.53	0.53	0.32

Maximized log-likelihood = −283.08.
[a] Estimated standard error of $\hat{b}$.
[b] Estimated significance level for testing the hypothesis b = 0.

dose-response problem. Although the use of the term effect modifier is an historical fact, and is unlikely to disappear quickly from the epidemiological literature, *Breslow and Day* [1980] indicate that 'the term is not a particularly happy one however'.

It is wise to regard most regression models as convenient, empirical descriptions of particular data sets. An interaction effect is a concept which only has meaning within the context of a particular model. If an interaction is identified, the aim of subsequent analyses, which may involve alternative regression models, should be to understand the nature of the data and of the biological process which has resulted in the empirical description obtained.

For example, Table 16.4 adds two additional variables to the model summarized in Table 16.3. The variable X_1X_4 is an interaction term which

Table 16.5. The results of an odds ratio regression analysis of endometrial cancer incidence which models estrogen use with a continuous covariate (cf. Table 16.4); the analysis stratifies on baseline age

Risk factor	Regression variable	Definition	$\hat{b}$	SE[a]	Significance level[b]
Estrogen use	X_1	logarithm of (duration of use + 1)	0.98	0.13	<0.0001
Obesity	X_3	1 if weight greater than 160 lbs; 0 otherwise	0.67	0.33	0.04
Hypertension	X_4	1 if history of high blood pressure; 0 otherwise	0.45	0.31	0.15
Parity	X_5	1 if number of children 2 or greater; 0 otherwise	0.59	0.31	0.06
Interaction	$X_1 X_4$	1 if both X_1 and X_4 equal 1; 0 otherwise	−0.02	0.18	0.91

Maximized log-likelihood = −286.543.
[a] Estimated standard error of $\hat{b}$.
[b] Estimated significance level for testing the hypothesis b = 0.

is the product of X_1 and X_4; $X_1 X_4$ is 1 only if a woman is hypertensive and used estrogen for 1–8 years, and is zero otherwise. A second interaction term, $X_2 X_4$, identifies women who are hypertensive and who have used estrogen for more than 8 years ($X_2 X_4 = 1$).

According to the analysis summarized in Table 16.4, the coefficient associated with $X_1 X_4$ is significantly different from zero. Thus, estrogen use of 1–8 years would have an estimated odds ratio of exp(1.78) = 5.93 for non-hypertensive women and exp(1.78−1.04) = 2.10 for hypertensive women. This indicates that the effect of moderate estrogen exposure is modified by hypertensive status. Alternatively, if we adopt the approach described in §12.3, we can interpret this significant interaction as indicating that exp(1.78 + 0.60−1.04), the individual odds ratio associated with being hypertensive and a moderate duration estrogen user, is less than the product of the odds ratios associated with hypertension, i.e., exp(0.60), and estrogen use of 1–8 years, i.e., exp(1.78), separately. In any event, it appears that estrogen use of 1–8 years duration does not further increase a hypertensive woman's risk of endometrial cancer.

The arbitrary grouping of the duration of estrogen use which appears in Tables 16.3 and 16.4 may not provide the simplest empirical model. Table 16.5 presents a model where estrogen use is defined to be the logarithm of (estrogen duration use + 1); the constant value 1 is added to prevent infinite values of the covariate. This model fits the data of *Weiss* et al. [1979] as well as the model summarized in Table 16.4. That this is the case can be determined by comparing maximized log-likelihoods, a technique which was mentioned briefly at the end of chapter 13. The formal details of the assessment are a bit more complicated here. However, it can be seen that the analysis presented in Table 16.5 requires only one variable to model the effect of estrogen use, and the interaction between estrogen use and hypertension is no longer significant. Thus, an interaction which was present in one empirical description of the data need not appear in another.

16.6. Mantel-Haenszel Methodology

Historically, and for convenience, many epidemiological studies have concentrated on a binary exposure variable and examined its relationship to disease after adjustment for potential confounding variables. Therefore, the analysis of such studies has often been based on stratified 2×2 tables of the type discussed in chapter 5 and shown in Table 16.6.

In chapter 11 and in this chapter, we have indicated how logistic regression models can be used to estimate odds ratios from data of this type. However, the use of logistic regression models does require a reasonably sophisticated computer package, and simpler methods of estimation have a

Table 16.6. A 2×2 table summarizing the binary data for level i of a confounding factor

	Confounding factor level i		Total
	success	failure	
Group 1	a_i	$A_i - a_i$	A_i
Group 2	b_i	$B_i - b_i$	B_i
Total	r_i	$N_i - r_i$	N_i

long history of use. The most widely used estimate of ψ, the common odds ratio, based on stratified 2×2 tables is the Mantel-Haenszel estimate, for which the defining equation is

$$\widehat{\text{OR}}_{\text{MH}} = \frac{\sum\limits_{i=1}^{k} a_i(B_i - b_i)/N_i}{\sum\limits_{i=1}^{k} (A_i - a_i)b_i/N_i}, \tag{16.6}$$

where there are k distinct 2×2 tables of the type illustrated in Table 16.6. Although it may not be apparent from equation (16.6), this estimate is a weighted average of the individual odds ratios $\{a_i(B_i - b_i)\}/\{(A_i - a_i)b_i\}$ in the k 2×2 tables. For completeness, the weight for the ith table is $(A_i - a_i)b_i/N_i$ a quantity which approximates the inverse of the variance of the individual estimate of the odds ratio in the ith table when ψ is near 1. Note also that $\widehat{\text{OR}}_{\text{MH}}$ is easy to compute and is not affected by zeros in the tables. Research has shown that the statistical properties of this estimate compare very favourably with the corresponding properties of estimates which are based on logistic regression models.

In chapter 5, we introduced the summary χ^2 statistic for testing the independence of exposure and disease. In the epidemiological literature, this same statistic is often called the Mantel-Haenszel χ^2 statistic for testing the null hypothesis that the common odds ratio is equal to 1. Despite all its merits, the Mantel-Haenszel estimator has one serious drawback; there is no convenient, simple, and generally useful estimate of its variance. There is an extensive statistical literature concerning variance estimates for $\widehat{\text{OR}}_{\text{MH}}$. Perhaps the most useful estimate is one proposed by *Hauck* [1979] for use in situations when the number of tables would not increase if the study was larger. Its formula, which is still not all that simple, is

$$V = \widehat{\text{OR}}_{\text{MH}} \sum_{i=1}^{k} S_i^2/W_i$$

where $S_i = \dfrac{(A_i - a_i)b_i}{N_i}$ and $W_i = \left[\dfrac{1}{a_i + 1/2} + \dfrac{1}{A_i - a_i + 1/2} + \dfrac{1}{b_i + 1/2} + \dfrac{1}{B_i - b_i + 1/2} \right]^{-1}$.

The fraction $\frac{1}{2}$ is added to each of the denominators in W_i to avoid division by zero.

Because of its good statistical properties, the Mantel-Haenszel estimator of a common odds ratio, ψ, can be recommended for use by researchers with few resources for the complicated calculations of logistic regression.

However, readers should remember that an analysis which is based on a logistic regression model is equivalent to a Mantel-Haenszel analysis, and offers the additional generality and advantages of regression modelling.

16.7. Clinical Epidemiology

At the beginning of this chapter, we remarked that previous chapters were primarily concerned with clinical studies, whereas epidemiology concentrates on the incidence of disease. In recent years, there has been increasing interest in what has been called 'clinical epidemiology'.

There has been some variation, and some debate, as to the nature of clinical epidemiology. Indeed, some have argued that the term is unnecessary. The exposition of medical statistics in this book implicitly defines some opinions on clinical epidemiology, but we do not intend to pursue this point. We do however express some sympathy with the definition given by *Weiss* [1986].

Weiss argues that 'epidemiology per se is the study of variation in the occurrence of disease and of the reasons for that variation'. He defines clinical epidemiology in a parallel way as 'the study of variation in the *outcome* of illness and of the reasons for that variation'. Whatever one's reaction, semantically, to the term clinical epidemiology, the area of study defined by *Weiss* is of obvious importance. It is our hope that this book will be useful to readers who are interested in this area.

References

Armitage, P.: Statistical methods in medical research (Blackwell, Oxford 1971).

Berkson, J.; Gage, R.P.: Calculation of survival rates for cancer. Proc. Staff Meet. Mayo Clin. *25:* 270–286 (1950).

Breslow, N.E.; Day, N.E.: Statistical methods in cancer research, vol. 1, The analysis of case-control studies (IARC, Lyon 1980).

Cox, D.R.: Regression models and life-tables (with discussion). J. R. statist. Soc. B *34:* 187–220 (1972).

Cutler, S.J.; Ederer, F.: Maximum utilization of the life table method in analyzing survival. J. chronic Dis. *8:* 699–712 (1958).

Duncan, B.B.A.; Zaimi, F.; Newman, G.B.; Jenkins, J.G.; Aveling, W.: Effect of premedication on the induction dose of thiopentone in children. Anaesthesia *39:* 426–428 (1984).

Farewell, V.T.; D'Angio, G.J.: A simulated study of historical controls using real data. Biometrics *37:* 169–176 (1981).

Fleming, T.R.; Harrington, D.P.; O'Brien, P.C.: Designs for group sequential tests. Controlled Clinical Trials *5:* 348–361 (1984).

Freedman, L.S.: Tables of the number of patients required in clinical trials using the logrank test. Statist. Med. *1:* 121–129 (1982).

Freireich, E.J.: The randomized clinical trial as an obstacle to clinical research; in Varco, Delaney, Controversy in surgery, vol. 2, pp. 5–12 (Saunders, Philadelphia 1983).

Gehan, E.A.: A generalized Wilcoxon test for comparing arbitrarily singly-censored samples. Biometrika *52:* 203–223 (1965).

Hauck, W.W.: The large sample variance of the Mantel-Haenszel estimator of a common odds ratio. Biometrics *35:* 817–819 (1979).

Irwin, J.O.: The place of mathematics in medical and biological statistics. J. R. statist. Soc. A *126:* 1–45 (1963).

Kaplan, E.L.; Meier, P.: Nonparametric estimation from incomplete observations. J. Am. statist. Ass. *53:* 457–481 (1958).

Lilienfeld, A.M.; Lilienfeld, D.E.: Foundations of epidemiology (Oxford University Press, New York 1980).

Mantle, M.J.; Greenwood, R.M.; Currey, H.L.F.: Backache in pregnancy. Rheumatol. Rehabil. *16:* 95–101 (1977).

McDonald, G.B.; Sharma, P.; Matthews, D.; Shulman, H.; Thomas, E.D.: Venocclusive disease of the liver after bone marrow transplantation: diagnosis, incidence and predisposing factors. Hepatology *4:* 116–122 (1984).

McPherson, K.: Statistics: the problem of examining accumulating data more than once. New Engl. J. Med. *290:* 501–502 (1974).

Medical Research Council: Treatment of pulmonary tuberculosis with streptomycin and para-amino-salicylic acid. Br. med. J. *ii:* 1073–1085 (1950).

Pearson, K.; Lee, A.: On the laws of inheritance in man. I. Inheritance of physical characters. Biometrika *2:* 357–462 (1903).

Peto, R.; Peto, J.: Asymptotically efficient rank invariant test procedures (with discussion). J. R. statist. Soc. A *135:* 185–206 (1972).

Peto, R.; Pike, M.C.; Armitage, P.; Breslow, N.E.; Cox, D.R.; Howard, S.V.; Mantel, N.; McPherson, K.; Peto, J.; Smith, P.G.: Design and analysis of randomized clinical trials requiring prolonged observation of each patient. I. Introduction and design. Br. J. Cancer *34:* 585–612 (1976).

Peto, R.; Pike, M.C.; Armitage, P.; Breslow, N.E.; Cox, D.R.; Howard, S.V.; Mantel, N.; McPherson, K.; Peto, J.; Smith, P.G.: Design and analysis of randomized clinical trials requiring prolonged observation of each patient. II. Analysis and examples. Br. J. Cancer *35:* 1–39 (1977).

Pocock, S.J.: Clinical trials, a practical approach (Wiley, Chichester 1983).

Prentice, R.L.; Kalbfleisch, J.D.; Peterson, A.V., Jr.; Flournoy, N.; Farewell, V.T.; Breslow, N.E.: The analysis of failure times in the presence of competing risks. Biometrics *34:* 541–554 (1978).

Prentice, R.L.; Marek, P.: A qualitative discrepancy between censored data rank tests. Biometrics *35:* 861–867 (1979).

Prentice, R.L.; Shimizu, Y.; Lin, C.H.; Peterson, A.V.; Kato, H.; Mason, M.W.; Szatrowski, T.P.: Serial blood pressure measurements and cardiovascular disease in a Japanese cohort. Am. J. Epidem. *116:* 1–28 (1982).

Sacks, H.; Chalmers, T.C.; Smith, H.: Randomized versus historical controls for clinical trials. Am. J. Med. *72:* 233–240 (1982).

Storb, R.; Prentice, R.L.; Thomas, E.D.: Marrow transplantation for treatment of aplastic anemia. New Engl. J. Med. *296:* 61–66 (1977).

Thomas, P.R.M.; Tefft, M.; D'Angio, G.J.; Norkool, P.; Farewell, V.T.: Relapse patterns in irradiated Second National Wilms' Tumor Study (NWTS-2) patients. Proc. Am. Soc. clin. Oncol. *24:* 69 (1983).

Wainwright, P.; Pelkman, C.; Wahlsten, D.: The relationship between nutritional effects on preweaning growth and behavioral development in mice. Dev. Psychobiol. (to appear 1988).

Weiss, N.S.: Clinical epidemiology: the study of the outcome of illness (Oxford University Press, New York 1986).

Weiss, N.S.; Szekeley, D.R.; English, D.R.; Schweid, A.J.: Endometrial cancer in relation to patterns of menopausal estrogen use. J. Am. med. Ass. *242:* 261–264 (1979).

Whitehead, J.: The design and analysis of sequential clinical trials (Ellis Horwood, Chichester 1983).

Yule, G.U.: The function of scientific method in scientific investigation. Industrial Fatigue Research Board Report *28:* 4 pp. (HMSO, London 1924).

Subject Index